DUKAN DIET 2025

110 New Tasty Recipes for Every Phase, Safe Weight Loss, Practical Tips for Sustainable Success

KLARLOCK

DISCLAIMER

Please note that the content of this book is based on personal experience and various sources of information. This book aims to provide useful and informative material on the topics covered in the publication. It is sold with the understanding that the author and publisher are not engaged in rendering any personal medical, health care, or other professional services in the book. The reader should consult his or her physician, health care provider, or other competent professional before adopting any suggestions in this book or drawing any conclusions. The author and publisher expressly disclaim responsibility for any liability, loss, or risk, personal or otherwise, arising, directly or indirectly, from the use and application of any contents of this book.

NOTE

In the context of this book, when we refer to "a cup" as a unit of measurement for ingredients, we mean using a standard kitchen cup with a capacity of approximately 2 milliliters. It is essential to use a measuring cup to get the right quantities of ingredients. If you don't have a measuring cup, you can use a graduated measuring cup, making sure to correctly correspond to the proportions indicated. Here are some examples 1 Cup of flour 100 gr. 1 cup of rice 200 gr. 1 Cup of Quinoa 200 g, It is recommended to level the dry ingredients in the cup using a spatula or the blade of a knife to obtain an accurate measurement. For liquid ingredients it is recommended to fill the cup to the brim without squeezing or leaving gaps.

TABLE OF CONTENT

CRUISE PHASE

CONSOLIDATION PHASE

109 WHOLE BREAD CROUTTONS WITH RICOTTA CREAM AND DRIED TOMATOES

111 CHICKEN SALAD WITH MANGO, AVOCADO AND SUNFLOWER SEEDS

STABILIZATION PHASE

113 GREEK SALAD WITH TOMATOES, CUCUMBERS, PEPPERS, OLIVES AND FETA

115 AVOCADO CARPACCIO WITH PRAWNS AND MANGO

117 WHOLE WHOLE BRUSCHETTE WITH TOMATOES, BASIL AND BUFFALO MOZZARELLA

119 WHOLE BREAD CANAPES WITH CHICKPEA HUMMUS AND GRILLED VEGETABLES

121 ROLLS OF RAW HAM WITH MELON AND FRESH CHEESE

123 QUINOA FRITTERS WITH SPINACH AND LIGHT CHEESE

125 TUNA SALAD WITH CANNELLINI BEANS, RED ONION AND PARSLEY

RECIPES FIRST DISHES

ATTACK PHASE

CRUISE PHASE

CONSOLIDATION PHASE

STABILIZATION PHASE

RECIPES SECOND DISHES

ATTACK PHASE

CRUISE PHASE

226 CHICKEN CURRY WITH GRILLED VEGETABLES

228 GRILLED SALMON WITH CITRUS SAUCE

230 BEEF STEAK WITH PEPPERS AND ONIONS

232 CHICKEN BREAST STUFFED WITH SPINACH AND SKINNY CHEESE

234 GRILLED TUNA WITH TOMATO AND BASIL SAUCE

236 COD IN PAPER WITH MIXED VEGETABLES

238 BAKED TURKEY WITH MEDITERRANEAN SPICES

240 VEAL MILANESE WITH MIXED SALAD

CONSOLIDATION PHASE

242 BAKED SALMON TROUT WITH POTATOES

244 VEGETABLE ROLLS WITH FETA AND TOMATOES

STABILIZATION PHASE

SIDE DISH RECIPES

ATTACK PHASE

CRUISE PHASE

285 BAKED AUBERGINES WITH TOMATO AND BASIL SAUCE

287 MIXED SALAD WITH CHICORY, LETTUCE, ROCKET AND GRATED CARROTS

CONSOLIDATION PHASE

289 COLD QUINOA WITH PEPPERS, TOMATOES AND BLACK OLIVES

291 BAKED SWEET POTATOES WITH ROSEMARY AND GARLIC

293 COURGETTE FLAN WITH RICOTTA AND EGGS

STABILIZATION PHASE

295 WHOLE WHOLE COUSCOUS WITH GRILLED VEGETABLES AND FRESH MINT

297 BAKED POTATOES WITH ROSEMARY AND GARLIC

299 MIXED VEGETABLE OMELETTE WITH SPINACH, TOMATOES AND COURGETTES

INTRODUCTION TO THE DUKAN DIET 2025

Welcome to the Dukan Diet 2025, an updated and comprehensive guide to achieving your weight loss and health goals through a scientifically proven and sustainable approach. Founded by Dr. Pierre Dukan in 1972, the Dukan Diet has gained popularity around the world for its effectiveness in promoting weight loss without sacrificing health or food satisfaction. Over the years, the Dukan Diet has been the subject of ongoing research and developments, adapting to the needs and latest scientific discoveries in the field of nutrition and health. In this 2025 edition, we will explore the fundamental principles of the Dukan Diet, its four distinctive phases, and strategies for long-term success.

Through the balance between lean proteins, vegetables, and the gradual replenishment of other foods, the Dukan Diet not only promotes weight loss, but also the building of healthy and sustainable eating habits. Each phase of the program is designed to offer a gradual, controlled progression, allowing your body to adapt and achieve lasting results. In this book, we will explore every aspect of the 2025 Dukan Diet in detail, providing practical advice, tips for success and testimonials from those who have embraced this approach and transformed their lives. Whether you are new to the Dukan Diet or want to deepen your knowledge, this book will be your reliable guide on your journey to a healthier and more fulfilling life. It is important to consult a doctor or dietician to have a personalized evaluation and to receive specific advice on the Dukan Diet.

WHAT IS THE DUKAN DIET

The Dukan diet is a high-protein diet created by the French doctor Pierre Dukan. The diet is divided into four phases:

Phase 1: Attack

This phase lasts 2 to 7 days and involves consuming unlimited lean proteins, such as meat, poultry, fish, eggs and tofu.

Image of Phase 1 Dukan Diet AttackOpens in a new window

Phase 1 Attack of the Dukan Diet

Vegetables are not allowed at this stage. The goal is to lose as much weight as possible in this phase.

Phase 2: Cruise

This phase lasts until you reach your desired weight.

In this phase, you alternate days of unlimited lean protein (PP days) with days where you can eat lean proteins and vegetables (PV days).

Phase 2 Dukan Diet Cruise

An example of a PP day is eating only grilled chicken, while an example of a PV day is eating grilled chicken with steamed vegetables. The goal is to continue losing weight, but at a slower pace.

Phase 3: Consolidation

This phase lasts 10 days for every pound lost during phase 2.

In this phase, carbohydrates, fruits and vegetables are gradually reintroduced. The goal is to prevent weight regain.

Phase 4: Stabilization

This phase lasts forever. At this stage, you can eat freely, but it is important to choose healthy foods and exercise regularly.

Phase 4 Stabilization of the Dukan Diet

The goal is to maintain the weight achieved.

Here are some of the potential benefits of the Dukan diet: Fast weight loss Improved glycemic control Reduced risk of cardiovascular disease Increased satiety Increased energy The Dukan diet is an effective way to lose weight, but it's important to be aware potential risks and side effects. The diet is high in protein and low in carbohydrates, which can lead to ketosis, a condition in which the body burns fat for energy instead of sugar. The diet is not suitable for everyone. People with medical conditions, such as kidney or liver disease, should not follow this diet. Pregnant or breastfeeding women should not follow this diet. It is important to consult a doctor before starting any new diet.

BENEFITS OF THE DUKAN DIET

The Dukan Diet offers a number of benefits for those who follow the program diligently. Here are some of the main benefits: 1. Rapid weight loss: The diet is designed to promote rapid weight loss, especially during the attack phase, in which it focuses on lean protein intake. 2. Reduced appetite: The high protein content of the diet can help reduce appetite and promote greater satiety, thus reducing the desire for excessive snacking. 3. Maintaining muscle mass: The diet focuses on protein intake, which is crucial for maintaining muscle mass during weight loss. 4. Structured Program: The diet is divided into four distinct phases, each with specific goals and clear guidelines, thus providing structure and planning for your weight loss journey.

5. Nutrition Education: The diet encourages food awareness and nutrient education, helping participants better understand the impact of foods on their health and weight. 6. Promotion of a healthy lifestyle: In addition to weight loss, the Dukan Diet also encourages the adoption of a healthy lifestyle through the consumption of nutritious foods, regular physical activity and long-term weight maintenance . 7. Community Support: Many people following the Dukan Diet find support and motivation through online communities and group meetings, which can help them stay motivated and share similar experiences with others. Always remember to consult a health professional before starting any diet program, including the Dukan Diet, to ensure it is safe and suitable for your individual needs.

THE FOUR PHASES OF THE DUKAN DIET

The Dukan Diet is divided into four distinct phases, each designed to achieve specific goals on your weight loss and maintenance journey. Here is an overview of the four phases of the Dukan Diet:

1. ATTACK PHASE:

This is the initial phase of the diet, during which you focus on eating only lean proteins for a limited period of time. The main goal of this phase is to quickly initiate weight loss by causing the body to burn excess fat. This attack phase usually lasts 2 to 7 days, depending on the weight to be lost and individual needs.

2. CRUISE PHASE:

During this phase, non-protein foods, such as vegetables, are gradually introduced to create a more balanced and sustainable diet over time. Alternate between protein-only days and protein-with-veggies days. This alternating cycle continues until you reach your desired weight. The duration of this phase depends on the amount of weight you want to lose.

3. CONSOLIDATION PHASE:

This phase aims to stabilize and consolidate the results obtained during the previous phases. During this phase, foods such as fruits, whole grain carbohydrates, cheeses, and extra portions of proteins and vegetables are gradually reintroduced. The duration of this phase is calculated based on the weight lost during the previous phases.

4. STABILIZATION PHASE:

This is the final phase of the diet, during which you learn to maintain the weight you have achieved in the long term. At this stage, there are no hard food restrictions, but it's important to follow some basic guidelines, such as having one protein-only day a week, eating three tablespoons of oat bran a day, and exercising regularly. The stabilization phase is designed to be followed throughout your life, maintaining a balance between your diet and healthy lifestyle. These four phases form the heart of the Dukan Diet, offering a structure and gradual progression to help people achieve their weight loss goals effectively and sustainably.

FOODS TO EAT AND FOODS TO AVOID

FOODS TO EAT ON THE DUKAN DIET

Attack Phase (1-7 days):

Unlimited lean protein: Meat (beef, veal, chicken, turkey, rabbit), fish (white, blue), eggs, tofu.

Vegetables not allowed.

Cruise Phase (variable):

Pure Protein (PP) Days: Unlimited lean protein as in the Attack Phase.

Protein and Vegetable Days (PV): Unlimited lean protein + Low-starch vegetables (spinach, chard, broccoli, cauliflower, cucumber, tomatoes).

Consolidation Phase (10 days per kg lost in Phase 2):

1 free meal per week: One meal with any food, in moderation.

2 days PP per week.

PV days with: 1 portion of fruit and 2 portions of wholemeal bread.

Stabilization Phase (forever):

Food freedom in moderation: Choose healthy and nutritious foods, limiting sugars, saturated fats and processed foods.

Examples of permitted foods:

Meat: Lean beef, veal, skinless chicken, turkey, rabbit, lean raw ham, bresaola.

Fish: White fish (cod, hake, plaice), blue fish (mackerel, sardines, salmon), crustaceans (prawns, scampi).

Eggs: Whole eggs, egg white.

Tofu: Natural tofu, silken tofu.

Low-starch vegetables: Spinach, chard, broccoli, cauliflower, cucumber, tomatoes, fennel, peppers, squash.

Fruit (Consolidation and Stabilization Phase): Apples, pears, strawberries, raspberries, oranges, grapefruits.

Wholemeal bread (Consolidation and Stabilization Phase): Wholemeal bread made from whole cereals, rye, oats.

Fats: Extra virgin olive oil, avocado, oily dried fruit (in moderation).

FOODS TO AVOID ON THE DUKAN DIET:

All phases:

Sugar and artificial sweeteners: Candy, biscuits, cakes, ice cream, sugary drinks.

Refined grains: White bread, pasta, rice, biscuits, crackers.

Legumes: Beans, chickpeas, lentils.

Fruit (Attack and Cruise Phase): Sugary fruit (bananas, grapes, figs), dried fruit.

Potatoes: White potatoes, sweet potatoes.

Fatty cheeses: Mature cheeses, spreadable cheeses.

Fatty cured meats: Salami, mortadella, bacon.

Alcoholic drinks: Wine, beer, spirits.

The complete list of permitted and prohibited foods in the Dukan Diet may vary depending on the phase and specific individual needs. Consulting a doctor or dietician is always advisable to adapt your food plan to your needs and ensure a safe and healthy approach to weight loss.

PLANNING MEALS WITH THE DUKAN DIET

Planning your meals is a key aspect of the success of the Dukan Diet. Planning your meals in advance helps you make healthy food choices, avoid temptation, and stay on course toward your weight loss goals. Here are some tips for planning meals on the Dukan Diet:

1. Choose your phase:

The first thing to do is determine what phase of the Dukan Diet you are in. This will affect your food choices and the structure of your meals.

2. Create a shopping list:

Once you know what foods are allowed in your current stage, create a detailed grocery list to ensure you have everything you need to prepare your meals.

3. Prepare meals in advance:

Set aside time on the weekend or in the evening to cook a few meals in advance. This will save you time during the week and help you stay on track with your diet.

4. Variety your choices:

While the Dukan Diet focuses on lean proteins and vegetables, it's important to vary your choices to avoid boredom and ensure you're getting all the nutrients you need.

EXAMPLES OF MEAL PLANS FOR THE DUKAN DIET:

Attack Phase (1-7 days):

Breakfast: Omelette with vegetables, Greek yogurt with oat bran, protein shake.

Lunch: Grilled chicken salad with vegetables, baked salmon with vegetables, omelette with vegetables.

Dinner: Lean beef steak with grilled vegetables, steamed cod with vegetables, sautéed tofu with vegetables.

Cruise Phase (variable):

Pure Protein (PP) Days: Same examples as the Attack Phase.

Protein and Vegetable (PV) Days: Add a serving of low-starch vegetables to each meal.

Consolidation Phase (10 days per kg lost in Phase 2):

Breakfast: Same examples as the Cruise Phase.

Lunch: Grilled chicken salad with vegetables and wholemeal bread, baked salmon with vegetables and wholemeal rice, omelette with vegetables and wholemeal bread.

Dinner: Lean beef steak with grilled vegetables and sweet potatoes, steamed cod with vegetables and quinoa, sautéed tofu with vegetables and brown rice.

Stabilization Phase (forever):

Breakfast: Greek yogurt with fruit and granola, scrambled eggs with vegetables and wholemeal bread, protein smoothie with fruit and vegetables.

Lunch: Grilled chicken salad with vegetables and wholemeal bread, baked salmon with vegetables and brown rice, quinoa with vegetables and tofu.

Dinner: Lean beef steak with grilled vegetables and sweet potatoes, steamed cod with vegetables and quinoa, sautéed tofu with vegetables and brown rice.

Remember that these are just examples and that it is important to tailor meal plans to your individual needs and preferences. Consulting a doctor or dietician can be helpful in creating a personalized and safe eating plan for you.

INCORPORATE EXERCISE INTO YOUR DUKAN DIET PLAN

Exercise is a critical component to the success of the Dukan Diet and maintaining a healthy weight over the long term. In addition to promoting weight loss, physical activity offers numerous health benefits, including:

Improved muscle tone and strength, Increased metabolism

Improved mood and energy levels

Greater sense of well-being and self-esteem

Here are some tips for incorporating exercise into your Dukan diet plan:

1. Choose activities you like:

Finding activities that you enjoy will make you more likely to stay active over time.

Try different options such as walking, running, swimming, cycling, dancing, yoga or team sports.

2. Start gradually:

If you're new to exercise, start with short sessions and gradually increase the duration and intensity over time.

3. Aim for 30 minutes of moderate physical activity most days of the week:

You can divide the activity into shorter sessions if necessary. For example, you can do three 10-minute sessions a day.

4. Include strength exercises:

You can use free weights, resistance bands, or your own body weight for strength exercises.

5. Listen to your body:

If you feel tired or sore, take a rest day or reduce the intensity of your workout.

6. Find a workout partner:

Working out with a friend or family member can be more fun and motivating.

7. Make exercise a part of your daily routine:

Find ways to incorporate physical activity into your day, such as taking the stairs instead of the elevator or parking further away from the store.

8. Don't give up: There will be days when you don't feel like working out, but it's important to persevere. The benefits of long-term exercise are worth the effort.

Specific exercises for the Dukan Diet:

Attack Phase (1-7 days): In this phase, focus on low-intensity activities such as slow walking, light swimming or yoga.

Cruise Phase (variable): Gradually increase the intensity and duration of your workouts. You can include activities like brisk walking, light running, cycling or strength training with light weights.

Consolidation Phase (10 days per kg lost in Phase 2): Continue with a regular exercise program that includes both cardio and strength training.

Stabilization Phase (forever): Maintain an active lifestyle with at least 30 minutes of moderate physical activity most days of the week.

A doctor or personal trainer can help you create a safe and effective exercise program for you. Incorporating exercise into your Dukan diet plan will help you achieve your weight loss goals and improve your overall health. Find activities you enjoy, start small, and gradually increase the intensity and duration of your workouts over time. Listen to your body, make exercise a part of your daily routine and don't give up!

TIPS FOR SUCCEEDING WITH THE DUKAN DIET

Following the Dukan Diet can be an effective way to lose weight, but it's important to do it in a healthy and safe way. Here are some tips to increase your chances of success with the Dukan Diet:

1. Consult your doctor:

Before starting the Dukan Diet, it is important to consult your doctor to make sure it is right for you. Your doctor can evaluate your health condition and give you personalized advice.

2. Follow the guidelines of each phase:

The Dukan Diet is divided into four phases, each with its own specific rules and restrictions. It is important to carefully follow the guidelines of each step to achieve the best results and reduce the risk of side effects.

3. Drink lots of water:

Drinking plenty of water is important for your overall health and is especially important during the Dukan Diet. Water helps keep your body hydrated, helps eliminate toxins and can reduce feelings of hunger.

4. Get enough fiber:

Fiber helps you feel full and aids digestion. The Dukan Diet includes a significant amount of protein, which can increase the risk of constipation. Taking fiber supplements or consuming foods rich in fiber, such as low-starch vegetables, can help prevent this problem.

5. Watch your salt intake:

A common side effect of the Dukan Diet is dehydration, which can lead to constipation and tiredness. It is important to reduce salt intake during your diet to avoid these problems.

6. Track your progress:

Tracking your weight and how you feel can help you stay motivated and gauge whether the diet is working for you.

7. Don't give up:

Weight loss takes time and effort. There will be days when you may feel discouraged, but it's important not to give up. Focus on your long-term goals and continue following your diet and exercise plan.

8. Search for support:

Having the support of friends, family, or an online group can help you stay on course and overcome challenges.

9. Listen to your body:

If you feel tired, weak, or have other negative side effects, it's important to listen to your body and rest or make changes to your eating plan.

10. Don't make the Dukan Diet a long-term lifestyle:

The Dukan Diet is a short-term weight loss program and is not meant to be followed forever. Once you reach your goal weight, it's important to transition to a healthy, balanced diet that includes a variety of nutritious foods.

By following these tips, you can increase your chances of success with the Dukan Diet and achieve your weight loss goals in a safe and healthy way.

SUCCESS STORIES AND TESTIMONIALS

The Dukan Diet has helped many people achieve their weight loss goals. Here are some success stories and testimonials from people who have had positive experiences with this diet:

1. Mary:

"I lost 20kg on the Dukan Diet and I feel better than ever! At first I was a little skeptical, but I decided to try it and I didn't regret it. I followed the guidelines carefully and have seen results ever since immediately. Not only did I lose weight, but I also have more energy and feel more confident in myself. I highly recommend the Dukan Diet to anyone who wants to lose weight in a healthy and safe way."

2. Mark:

"I had been overweight for years and had tried many diets without success. Then I discovered the Dukan Diet and finally found a diet that worked for me. I lost 15 kg in 3 months and maintained my new weight for over a year The Dukan Diet has taught me to make healthy food choices and have a healthier relationship with food.

3. Anna:

The Dukan Diet has helped me change my lifestyle and become a healthier and happier person. I lost 30 kg and gained more self-confidence. Now I like to exercise and cook healthy food. The Dukan Diet has been a turning point in my life and I wouldn't change it for the world."

4. Roberto:

"I was an emotional eater and often found myself comforting myself with food. The Dukan Diet helped me identify my emotional triggers and develop healthier strategies for coping with stress. I lost 20 pounds and learned to eat to nourish my body, not my emotions. The Dukan Diet gave me the tools I needed to change my relationship with food and improve my mental health."

5. Laura:

"I followed the Dukan Diet to prepare for my wedding and I couldn't have asked for anything better! I lost 8kg in 2 months and felt beautiful in my wedding dress. The Dukan Diet gave me the energy and confidence I needed I needed to fully enjoy my special day. I highly recommend the Dukan Diet to all brides who want to feel their best on their most important day."

It is important to note that these are just some testimonials and that individual results may vary. The Dukan Diet can be an effective way to lose weight for many people, but it's important to follow the guidelines carefully and listen to your body. Consulting a doctor or dietician before starting any diet, particularly if you have pre-existing medical conditions, is always advisable.

TIPS FOR MAINTAINING LONG-TERM SUCCESS

Achieving your weight loss goals on the Dukan Diet is a fantastic achievement, but maintaining long-term success requires commitment and proper strategies. Here are some tips that can help you keep the weight off and maintain a healthy lifestyle:

1. Gradually move to the Stabilization Phase:

Once you reach your goal weight, don't immediately switch to a free diet. Make a gradual transition to the Stabilization Phase, slowly reintroducing foods allowed in previous phases in moderation. This will help your body adapt to the new diet and reduce the risk of gaining weight back quickly.

2. Listen to your body:

Pay attention to your body's signals and adjust your diet accordingly. If you notice weight gain or feel tired or lacking energy, you may need to make changes to your eating plan or exercise program.

3. Maintain regular physical activity:

Exercise is key to maintaining a healthy weight and improving overall health. Aim to do at least 30 minutes of moderate physical activity most days of the week. You can include a variety of activities such as walking, running, swimming, cycling or strength training.

4. Make healthy food choices:

Even if you are no longer in the active phase of the Dukan Diet, it is important to continue making healthy food choices. Limit your intake of processed foods, added sugars and saturated fats.

5. Pay attention to portions:

Even if you're eating healthy foods, it's important to pay attention to portion sizes to avoid taking in too many calories. Use smaller plates, measure portions and be careful not to eat too quickly.

6. Plan meals and shop in advance:

Planning meals in advance and shopping with a list can help you make healthy food choices and avoid making impulsive purchases at the supermarket.

7. Find your support:

Having the support of friends, family can help you stay motivated and on track. Sharing your goals and challenges with others can be helpful and encouraging.

8. Don't be discouraged if you have setbacks:

It's normal to have some hiccups from time to time.

If you lose weight or gain some weight back, don't be discouraged. Simply get back on track and continue pursuing your long-term goals.

9. Track your progress:

Continuing to monitor your weight and how you feel can help you stay motivated and identify any areas where you may need to make changes to your lifestyle.

10. Reward yourself:

Celebrate your successes along the way! Rewarding yourself for achieving your goals can help you stay motivated and make maintaining a healthy lifestyle more enjoyable.

Remember that maintaining long-term success with the Dukan Diet or any other weight loss program requires commitment and consistency. However, with the right strategies and the right mindset, you can achieve your goals and enjoy a healthier, happier life.

CONCLUSION: ADOPT A HEALTHIER LIFESTYLE BY FOLLOWING THE DUKAN DIET

The Dukan Diet can be an effective way to lose weight and improve overall health, if followed correctly. However, it is important to remember that it is not a miracle solution and requires commitment and consistency to achieve lasting results.

Here are some key points to consider:

The Dukan Diet is a short-term weight loss program and is not meant to be followed forever. Once you reach your goal weight, it's important to transition to a healthy, balanced diet that includes a variety of nutritious foods. If you're thinking about following the Dukan Diet, it's important to talk to your doctor to make sure it's right for you. A doctor or dietician can help you create a personalized plan that is safe and effective for you.

In addition to following the Dukan Diet, it is important to adopt a healthier lifestyle to maintain long-term success. This includes:

Do regular physical activity

Make healthy food choices

Pay attention to portions

Plan meals and shop in advance

Find your support

Monitor progress

Reward yourself

Don't be discouraged if you have some setbacks

Adopting a healthier lifestyle can help you achieve your weight loss goals and improve your overall health and well-being.

FUTURE PROSPECTS FOR THE DUKAN DIET

The Dukan Diet is a popular weight loss program that has been around for over 20 years. Over the years, the diet has undergone several changes and a lot of research has been conducted on its effects on health.

Here are some future prospects for the Dukan Diet:

Continuing Research: More research is likely to be conducted on the health effects of the Dukan Diet, both in the short and long term. This research could help identify the potential benefits and risks of the diet and determine who it is best suited for.

Customization: As technology advances, it is possible that the Dukan Diet may be further customized to meet individual needs. This may involve using genetic testing or other biomarkers to determine the optimal eating plan for each person.

Integration with technology: The Dukan Diet may be integrated with technology such as smartphone apps or wearable devices to help people follow the diet and monitor their progress.

New variations of the diet: New variations of the Dukan Diet may be developed that are based on the original principles but take into account new research or dietary trends.

It is important to note that these are only future prospects and it is not possible to predict with certainty what the future holds for the Dukan Diet. However, it is clear that the diet will continue to evolve as new research is conducted and technologies evolve.

Regardless of the future of the Dukan Diet, it's important to remember that there is no silver bullet to weight loss. The best way to lose weight and keep it off is to eat a healthy, balanced diet and exercise regularly.

Additionally, it is always important to consult your doctor before starting any new weight loss program, particularly if you have pre-existing medical conditions.

RECIPES APPETIZERS

STUFFED EGGS WITH TUNA AND PARSLEY

Preparation time: 15 minutes

Cooking time: 10 minutes

Doses: 1 person

Ingredients:

1 egg

1 can of natural tuna (80 g)

1 tablespoon chopped parsley

1 tablespoon Greek yogurt

1/2 clove garlic, minced (optional)

Salt and Pepper To Taste

Preparation:

Cook the egg in boiling water for 10 minutes. Drain it and cool it under cold running water. Peel the egg and cut it in half lengthwise. Remove the yolk and place it in a bowl. Mash the egg yolk with a fork. Add the tuna, parsley, yogurt, garlic (if using), salt and pepper. Mix well until a homogeneous mixture is obtained. Fill the egg cavities with the tuna mixture. Serve immediately or store in the refrigerator for up to 2 days.

Nutritional values (per serving):

Calories: 150 kcal

Protein: 15 gr

Fat: 8 gr

Carbohydrates: 2 gr

BEEF CARPACCIO WITH ARUGULA AND PARMESAN FLAKES

Preparation time: 10 minutes

Cooking time: 0 minutes

Doses: 1 person

Ingredients:

100g of beef

lean (e.g. fillet, silverside)

50 g of Arugula

20 g of parmesan flakes

Extra virgin olive oil to taste

Lemon juice to taste

Salt and Pepper To Taste

Preparation:

Thinly slice the beef with a sharp knife or slicer. Arrange the slices of meat on a serving plate. Season with extra virgin olive oil, lemon juice, salt and pepper. Add the Arugula and parmesan flakes. Serve immediately.

Nutritional values (per serving):

Calories: 250 kcal

Protein: 25 gr

Fat: 15 gr

Carbohydrates: 1 g

GRILLED PRAWNS SKEWERS WITH LEMON

Preparation time: 10 minutes

Cooking time: 5-7 minutes

Doses: 1 person

Ingredients:

100g of cleaned fresh prawns

1/2 lemon

1/2 tablespoon of oil

extra virgin olive oil

Salt and Pepper To Taste

Preparation:

Wash the prawns and dry them with absorbent paper. Thread the prawns onto a wooden skewer. Drizzle the prawns with extra virgin olive oil, salt and pepper. Grill the shrimp for 5-7 minutes per side, or until golden brown and cooked through. Serve the shrimp with lemon wedges.

Nutritional values (per serving):

Calories: 125 kcal

Protein: 15 gr

Fat: 5 gr

Carbohydrates: 0 gr

CHICKEN SALAD WITH CELERY AND MUSTARD

Preparation time: 15 minutes

Cooking time: 20 minutes

Doses: 1 person

Ingredients:

150g of chicken breast

grilled or boiled

1 stalk of celery

1 tablespoon Greek yogurt

1 teaspoon of

Dijon mustard

Salt and Pepper To Taste

Preparation:

Cut the chicken breast into cubes. Wash the celery and cut it into thin slices. In a bowl, mix the chicken, celery, yogurt, mustard, salt and pepper. Serve the salad immediately. You can add other ingredients to the salad, such as tomatoes, cucumbers or olives. You can prepare the salad in advance and store it in the refrigerator for up to 2 days.

Nutritional values (per serving):

Calories: 300 kcal

Protein: 35 gr

Fat: 15 gr

Carbohydrates: 5 gr

SMOKED SALMON CANAPES WITH CUCUMBER

Preparation time: 5 minutes

Cooking time: 0 minutes

Doses: 1 person

Ingredients:

1 slice of wholemeal bread

50 g of smoked salmon

1/4 of a cucumber

Chopped parsley (optional)

Salt and Pepper To Taste

Preparation:

Toast wholemeal bread. Arrange the smoked salmon on the bread. Slice the cucumber thinly and arrange it on the salmon. Sprinkle with chopped parsley (optional). Salt and pepper to taste.

Nutritional values (per serving):

Calories: 250 kcal

Protein: 25 gr

Fat: 12 gr

Carbohydrates: 5 gr

GRILLED COURGETTES WITH FRESH TOMATO SAUCE

Preparation time: 15 minutes

Cooking time: 10 minutes

Doses: 1 person

Ingredients:

1 medium courgette

1 ripe tomato

1 tablespoon of oil

extra virgin olive oil

Chopped fresh basil

Salt and Pepper To Taste

Preparation:

Wash the courgette and cut it into slices about 1 cm thick. Grill the courgettes for 5-7 minutes per side, or until golden and soft. In the meantime, prepare the tomato sauce: cut the tomato into small pieces and place it in a bowl. Add the extra virgin olive oil, chopped basil, salt and pepper. Mix well. Serve the grilled courgettes with the fresh tomato sauce. You can add other ingredients to the tomato sauce, such as onion, garlic or chili pepper. If you prefer, you can cook the courgettes in the oven instead of on the grill.

Nutritional values (per serving):

Calories: 150 kcal

Protein: 10 gr

Fat: 8 gr

Carbohydrates: 5 gr

TOMATOES STUFFED
OF RICOTTA AND BASIL

Preparation time: 15 minutes

Cooking time: 15 minutes

Doses: 1 person

Ingredients:

10 cherry tomatoes

50 g of ricotta

1 tablespoon basil

fresh chopped

Salt and Pepper To Taste

Extra virgin olive oil

olive (optional)

Preparation:

Wash the cherry tomatoes and cut them in half lengthwise. Remove the seeds and pulp from the cherry tomatoes with a teaspoon. In a bowl, mix the ricotta, chopped basil, salt and pepper. Fill the cherry tomatoes with the ricotta mixture. Drizzle the cherry tomatoes with extra virgin olive oil (optional). Cook the cherry tomatoes in a preheated oven at 180°C for 15 minutes, or until they are golden.

Nutritional values (per serving):

Calories: 150 kcal

Protein: 15 gr

Fat: 8 gr

Carbohydrates: 5 gr

ROASTED PEPPERS STUFFED WITH TUNA AND CAPERS

Preparation time: 20 minutes

Cooking time: 30 minutes

Doses: 1 person

Ingredients:

1 red pepper

50 g of natural tuna

1 tablespoon capers

1 tablespoon of oil

extra virgin olive oil

Chopped parsley (optional)

Salt and Pepper To Taste

Preparation:

Wash the pepper and cut it in half lengthwise. Remove the seeds and the white part of the pepper. Cook the peppers in a preheated oven at 180°C for 30 minutes, or until they are soft. In the meantime, prepare the filling: in a bowl, crumble the tuna, add the capers, extra virgin olive oil, chopped parsley (optional), salt and pepper. Mix well. When the peppers are cooked, stuff them with the tuna mixture. Serve the peppers hot or cold. You can add other ingredients to the filling, such as olives, dried tomatoes or onion. Nutritional values (per serving):

Calories: 250 kcal

Protein: 25 gr

Fat: 15 gr

Carbohydrates: 5 gr

MOZZARELLA AND TOMATOES SKEWERS

Preparation time: 10 minutes

Cooking time: 0 minutes

Doses: 1 person

Ingredients:

5 cherry tomatoes

5 morsels of mozzarella

Fresh basil (optional)

Extra virgin olive oil

olive (optional)

Salt and Pepper To Taste

Preparation:

Wash the cherry tomatoes and cut them in half. Drain the mozzarella and cut it into cubes. Thread the cherry tomatoes and mozzarella cubes alternately onto a wooden skewer. Decorate with fresh basil leaves (optional). Drizzle with extra virgin olive oil (optional). Salt and pepper to taste. You can use cherry tomatoes of different varieties and colors to make the skewers more colorful. If you prefer, you can use light or low-fat mozzarella.

Nutritional values (per serving):

Calories: 200 kcal

Protein: 20 gr

Fat: 12 gr

Carbohydrates: 5 gr

CHICKEN SALAD WITH GRILLED VEGETABLES

Preparation time: 20 minutes

Cooking time: 15 minutes

Doses: 1 person

Ingredients:

150g of chicken breast

grilled or boiled

1 medium courgette

1 medium aubergine

1 red pepper

1 tablespoon of oil

extra virgin olive oil

Chopped fresh basil

Salt and Pepper To Taste

Preparation:

Wash the vegetables and cut them into slices. Grill vegetables for 5-7 minutes per side, or until golden and soft. Cut the chicken breast into cubes. In a bowl, mix the chicken, grilled vegetables, extra virgin olive oil, chopped basil, salt and pepper. Serve the salad immediately.

Nutritional values (per serving):

Calories: 350 kcal

Protein: 40 gr

Fat: 15 gr

Carbohydrates: 10 gr

SMOKED SALMON MOUSSE WITH GREEK YOGURT

79

Preparation time: 10 minutes

Cooking time: 0 minutes

Doses: 1 person

Ingredients:

50 g of smoked salmon

100g of Greek yogurt

1 tablespoon lemon juice

Chives

chopped (optional)

Salt and Pepper To Taste

Preparation:

Blend the smoked salmon, Greek yogurt, lemon juice, salt and pepper in a blender until smooth. Decorate with chopped chives (optional). Serve the mousse immediately. You can use other types of smoked fish, such as trout or mackerel. If you prefer, you can use low-fat or light Greek yogurt. You can add other ingredients to the mousse, such as avocado, cream cheese or spices

Nutritional values (per serving):

Calories: 250 kcal

Protein: 30 gr

Fat: 12 gr

Carbohydrates: 5 gr

BEET CARPACCIO WITH RICOTTA

Preparation time: 15 minutes

Cooking time: 0 minutes

Doses: 1 person

Ingredients:

100 g of pre-cooked beetroot

50 g of ricotta

1 walnut

Chopped parsley

(optional)

Salt and Pepper To Taste

Extra virgin olive oil

olive (optional)

Preparation:

Peel the pre-cooked beetroot and cut it into thin slices with a mandolin or sharp knife. Arrange the beetroot slices on a serving plate. Crumble the ricotta over the beetroot slices. Chop the walnut and sprinkle it on the ricotta. Sprinkle with chopped parsley (optional). Salt and pepper to taste. Drizzle with extra virgin olive oil (optional).

Nutritional values (per serving):

Calories: 250 kcal

Protein: 20 gr

Fat: 15 gr

Carbohydrates: 10 gr

SHRIMP AND COURGETTE SKEWERS

Preparation time: 20 minutes

Cooking time: 10 minutes

Doses: 1 person

Ingredients:

100g of cleaned fresh prawns

1 medium courgette

1 tablespoon of oil

extra virgin olive oil

Chopped fresh basil

Salt and Pepper To Taste

Preparation:

Wash the prawns and dry them with absorbent paper. Wash the courgette and cut it into rounds. Thread the prawns and courgette slices alternately onto a wooden skewer. Drizzle the skewers with extra virgin olive oil, salt and pepper. Grill the skewers for 5-7 minutes per side, or until the prawns are golden brown and cooked through. Decorate with chopped fresh basil. You can use other types of vegetables for the skewers, such as peppers, eggplant or onions. If you prefer, you can cook the skewers in the oven instead of on the grill.

Nutritional values (per serving):

Calories: 300 kcal

Protein: 35 gr

Fat: 15 gr

Carbohydrates: 5 gr

STUFFED EGGS WITH TUNA AND GREEK YOGURT

Preparation time: 15 minutes

Cooking time: 10 minutes

Doses: 1 person

Ingredients:

2 eggs

50 g of natural tuna

2 tablespoons Greek yogurt

1 tablespoon capers

Parsley

chopped (optional)

Salt and Pepper To Taste

Preparation:

Cook the eggs in boiling water for 10 minutes. Drain them and cool them under cold water. Peel the eggs and cut them in half lengthwise. Remove the egg yolks and place them in a bowl. Chop the tuna and add it to the egg yolks. Add the Greek yogurt, capers, chopped parsley (optional), salt and pepper. Mix well. Fill the egg cavities with the tuna mixture. Serve immediately.

Nutritional values (per serving):

Calories: 250 kcal

Protein: 25 gr

Fat: 15 gr

Carbohydrates: 5 gr

SEAFOOD SALAD WITH VEGETABLES

Preparation time: 20 minutes

Cooking time: 10 minutes

Doses: 1 person

Ingredients:

100g of cleaned fresh prawns

100g of calamari

1 medium courgette

1 tomato

1 tablespoon of oil

extra virgin olive oil

Chopped fresh basil

Salt and Pepper To Taste

Preparation:

Wash the prawns and squid and dry them with absorbent paper. Cook the prawns and calamari in boiling water for 5 minutes. Drain them and cool them. Wash the courgette and cut it into thin slices. Cut the tomato into small pieces. In a bowl, mix the prawns, calamari, courgette, tomato, extra virgin olive oil, chopped basil, salt and pepper. Serve the salad immediately.You can use other types of fish and seafood for the salad. If you prefer, you can cook the shrimp and calamari on the grill or steam instead of boiling water.

Nutritional values (per serving):

Calories: 350 kcal

Protein: 40 gr

Fat: 15 gr

Carbohydrates: 10 gr

SALMON CARPACCIO WITH YOGURT AND CHIVES SAUCE

Preparation time: 15 minutes

Cooking time: 0 minutes

Doses: 1 person

Ingredients:

100g of smoked salmon

100g of Greek yogurt

1 tablespoon lemon juice

1 tablespoon chopped chives

Salt and Pepper To Taste

Preparation:

Arrange the smoked salmon slices on a serving plate. In a bowl, mix the Greek yogurt, lemon juice, chopped chives, salt and pepper. Pour the yogurt sauce over the smoked salmon. Serve immediately.

Nutritional values (per serving):

Calories: 300 kcal

Protein: 35 gr

Fat: 15 gr

Carbohydrates: 5 gr

COURGETTE FRITTERS WITH MINT AND LEMON

Preparation time: 20 minutes

Cooking time: 10 minutes

Doses: 1 person

Ingredients:

1 medium 1 egg

2 tablespoons oat flour

1 tablespoon chopped fresh mint

1 tablespoon lemon juice

Salt and Pepper To Taste

Extra virgin olive oil

olive for frying

Preparation:

Wash the courgette and grate it. In a bowl, mix the grated courgette, egg, oat flour, chopped mint, lemon juice, salt and pepper. Heat the extra virgin olive oil in a non-stick pan. Pour a spoonful of pancake mixture into the pan and cook for 2-3 minutes per side, or until golden brown. Drain the pancakes on absorbent paper. Serve immediately.

Nutritional values (per serving):

Calories: 250 kcal

Protein: 15 gr

Fat: 15 gr

Carbohydrates: 15 gr

PEPPER ROLLS WITH TUNA AND BLACK OLIVES

93

Preparation time: 25 minutes

Cooking time: 15 minutes

Doses: 1 person

Ingredients:

1 red pepper

50 g of natural tuna

10 black olives

1 tablespoon capers

1 tablespoon of

chopped parsley

Salt and Pepper To Taste

Extra virgin olive oil

olive (optional)

Preparation:

Wash the pepper and cut it into strips about 2 cm wide. Cook the pepper strips in boiling water for 5 minutes. Drain them and cool them. Chop the tuna and mix it with the black olives, capers, chopped parsley, salt and pepper. Place a spoonful of tuna mixture on each pepper strip. Roll the pepper strips to form rolls. Drizzle the rolls with extra virgin olive oil (optional). Serve immediately. You can add other ingredients to the tuna mixture, such as cream cheese or spices.

Nutritional values (per serving):

Calories: 350 kcal

Protein: 35 gr

Fat: 20 gr

Carbohydrates: 5 gr

QUINOA SALAD WITH GRILLED VEGETABLES AND FETA

Preparation time: 30 minutes

Cooking time: 20 minutes

Doses: 1 person

Ingredients:

50g of quinoa

1 medium courgette

1 medium aubergine

1 red pepper

50 g of feta

1 tablespoon of oil

extra virgin olive oil

Chopped fresh basil

Salt and Pepper To Taste

Preparation:

Rinse the quinoa under running water. Cook the quinoa in boiling salted water for 15 minutes. Drain it and cool it. Wash the vegetables and cut them into slices. Grill vegetables for 5-7 minutes per side, or until golden and soft. Cut the feta into cubes. In a bowl, mix the quinoa, grilled vegetables, feta, extra virgin olive oil, chopped basil, salt and pepper. Serve the salad immediately.

Nutritional values (per serving):

Calories: 450 kcal

Protein: 30 gr

Fat: 20 gr

Carbohydrates: 35 gr

WHOLE WHOLE BRUSCHETTE WITH TOMATOES AND FRESH BASIL

Preparation time: 15 minutes

Cooking time: 10 minutes

Doses: 4 bruschettas

Ingredients:

4 slices of wholemeal bread

200g of cherry tomatoes

10 fresh basil leaves

1 clove of garlic

2 tablespoons of oil

extra virgin olive oil

Salt and Pepper To Taste

Preparation:

Cut the cherry tomatoes into small pieces. Chop the fresh basil. Fry the chopped garlic in extra virgin olive oil for 1 minute. Add the cherry tomatoes and cook for 5 minutes. Salt and pepper to taste. Toast the slices of wholemeal bread. Spread the bread slices with the cherry tomato mixture. Decorate with fresh basil leaves. Serve the bruschetta immediately. You can use other types of vegetables for the bruschetta, such as peppers, aubergines or onions.

Nutritional values (per serving):

Calories: 250 kcal

Protein: 10 gr

Fat: 15 gr

Carbohydrates: 25 gr

CAPRESE WITH TOMATO, LIGHT MOZZARELLA AND BASIL

Preparation time: 10 minutes

Cooking time: 0 minutes

Doses: 1 person

Ingredients:

1 ripe tomato

100g of light mozzarella

5 fresh basil leaves

Extra virgin olive oil

olive (optional)

Salt and Pepper To Taste

Preparation:

Wash the tomato and cut it into slices. Cut the light mozzarella into slices. Arrange the tomato and mozzarella slices on a plate alternating them. Decorate with fresh basil leaves. Drizzle with extra virgin olive oil (optional). Salt and pepper to taste. Serve the caprese immediately.

Nutritional values (per serving):

Calories: 250 kcal

Protein: 25 gr

Fat: 15 gr

Carbohydrates: 5 gr

WHOLE BREAD CANAPÉS INTEGRAL WITH AVOCADO AND SMOKED SALMON

Preparation time: 15 minutes

Cooking time: 0 minutes

Servings: 2 canapés

Ingredients:

2 slices of wholemeal bread

1/2 ripe avocado

50 g of smoked salmon

Lemon juice (optional)

Salt and Pepper To Taste

Preparation:

Toast the slices of wholemeal bread. Mash the avocado with a fork and spread it on the toast. Arrange the smoked salmon on the bread with the avocado. Drizzle with lemon juice (optional). Salt and pepper to taste. Serve the canapés immediately. You can use other types of bread for canapés, such as rye bread or cereal bread. If you prefer, you can bake the avocado for 10 minutes before mashing it.

Nutritional values (per serving):

Calories: 350 kcal

Protein: 30 gr

Fat: 20 gr

Carbohydrates: 20 gr

BUCKWHEAT FRITTERS WITH COURGETTES AND PARMESAN

Preparation time: 20 minutes

Cooking time: 10 minutes

Servings: 4 pancakes

Ingredients:

50 g of buckwheat flour

1 medium courgette

30 g of grated parmesan

1 egg

1 tablespoon of skimmed milk

1 tablespoon of oil

extra virgin olive oil

Salt and Pepper To Taste

Preparation:

Wash the courgette and grate it. In a bowl, mix the buckwheat flour, grated parmesan, egg, skimmed milk, extra virgin olive oil, salt and pepper. Add the grated courgette and mix well. Heat the extra virgin olive oil in a non-stick pan. Pour a spoonful of pancake mixture into the pan and cook for 2-3 minutes per side, or until golden brown. Drain the pancakes on absorbent paper. Serve the pancakes immediately.

Nutritional values (per serving):

Calories: 250 kcal

Protein: 15 gr

Fat: 15 gr

Carbohydrates: 20 gr

LENTIL SALAD WITH ROASTED PEPPERS AND TUNA

Preparation time: 30 minutes

Cooking time: 20 minutes

Doses: 1 person

Ingredients:

50 g of dried lentils

1 red pepper

50 g of natural tuna

1 tablespoon of oil

extra virgin olive oil

Red onion (optional)

Chopped parsley (optional)

Salt and Pepper To Taste

Preparation:

Rinse the lentils under running water. Cook the lentils in boiling salted water for 20 minutes. Drain them and cool them. Wash the pepper and cut it into strips. Bake or grill the pepper strips for 10 minutes, or until soft. Chop the tuna. In a bowl, mix the lentils, roasted peppers, tuna, extra virgin olive oil, salt and pepper. Add chopped red onion and chopped parsley (optional). Serve the salad immediately. You can use other types of legumes for the salad, such as chickpeas or beans.

Nutritional values (per serving):

Calories: 400 kcal

Protein: 35 gr

Fat: 20 gr

Carbohydrates: 25 gr

GRILLED AUBERGINES ROLLS WITH COOKED HAM AND LIGHT CHEESE

Preparation time: 25 minutes

Cooking time: 15 minutes

Doses: 2 rolls

Ingredients:

1 medium aubergine

50 g of cooked ham

50 g of light cheese

Fresh basil (optional)

Extra virgin olive oil

olive (optional)

Salt and Pepper To Taste

Preparation:

Wash the aubergine and cut it into thin longitudinal slices. Grill the aubergine slices for 5 minutes per side, or until soft. Drain them and cool them. Arrange a slice of cooked ham on each slice of grilled aubergine. Add a slice of light cheese. Roll up the aubergine slices to form rolls. Decorate with fresh basil (optional). Drizzle with extra virgin olive oil (optional). Salt and pepper to taste. Serve the rolls immediately.

Nutritional values (per serving):

Calories: 300 kcal

Protein: 25 gr

Fat: 15 gr

Carbohydrates: 10 gr

WHOLE WHOLE BREAD CROUTTONS WITH RICOTTA CREAM AND DRIED TOMATOES

Preparation time: 15 minutes

Cooking time: 0 minutes

Servings: 4 croutons

Ingredients:

4 slices of wholemeal bread

100 g of ricotta

5 dried tomatoes

Fresh basil (optional)

Extra virgin olive oil

olive (optional)

Salt and Pepper To Taste

Preparation:

Toast the slices of wholemeal bread. In a bowl, mix the ricotta, chopped dried tomatoes, chopped fresh basil (optional), extra virgin olive oil (optional), salt and pepper. Spread the ricotta cream on the wholemeal bread croutons. Serve the croutons immediately.

Nutritional values (per serving):

Calories: 250 kcal

Protein: 15 gr

Fat: 15 gr

Carbohydrates: 20 gr

CHICKEN SALAD WITH MANGO, AVOCADO AND SUNFLOWER SEEDS

Preparation time: 20 minutes

Cooking time: 10 minutes (for chicken)

Doses: 1 person

Ingredients:

100g of chicken breast

1/2 ripe mango

1/2 ripe avocado

1 tablespoon sunflower seeds

Lime juice (optional)

Extra virgin olive oil

olive (optional)

Salt and Pepper To Taste

Preparation:

Cook the chicken breast on the grill or in a pan for 10 minutes. Cut the chicken into small pieces. Cut the mango into small pieces. Cut the avocado into small pieces. In a bowl, mix the chicken, mango, avocado, sunflower seeds, lime juice (optional), extra virgin olive oil (optional), salt and pepper. Serve the salad immediately. You can use other fruits for the salad, such as pineapple or papaya. If you prefer, you can cook the chicken in the oven. Nutritional values (per portion):

Calories: 450 kcal

Protein: 35 gr

Fat: 25 gr

Carbohydrates: 15 gr

GREEK SALAD WITH TOMATOES, CUCUMBERS, PEPPERS, OLIVES AND FETA

Preparation time: 20 minutes

Cooking time: 0 minutes

Doses: 1 person

Ingredients:

1 ripe tomato

1/2 cucumber

1/2 green or red pepper

10 black olives

50 g of feta

1 tablespoon extra virgin olive oil

Fresh oregano (optional)

Salt and Pepper To Taste

Preparation:

Wash the tomato, cucumber and pepper. Cut the tomato into slices, the cucumber into pieces and the pepper into strips. Arrange the vegetables on a serving plate. Add the black olives and crumbled feta. Drizzle with extra virgin olive oil. Sprinkle with fresh oregano (optional). Salt and pepper to taste. Serve the salad immediately.

Nutritional values (per serving):

Calories: 350 kcal

Protein: 25 gr

Fat: 20 gr

Carbohydrates: 10 gr

AVOCADO CARPACCIO WITH PRAWNS AND MANGO

Preparation time: 20 minutes

Cooking time: 0 minutes

Doses: 1 person

Ingredients:

1/2 ripe avocado

5 cleaned prawns

1/2 ripe mango

1 tablespoon lime juice

1 tablespoon of oil

extra virgin olive oil

Sesame seeds (optional)

Salt and Pepper To Taste

Preparation:

Cut the avocado into thin slices. Arrange the avocado slices on a serving plate. Chop the prawns and arrange them on the avocado. Cut the mango into thin slices and arrange them on the prawns. Drizzle with lime juice and extra virgin olive oil. Sprinkle with sesame seeds (optional). Salt and pepper to taste. Serve the carpaccio immediately.

Nutritional values (per serving):

Calories: 400 kcal

Protein: 30 gr

Fat: 25 gr

Carbohydrates: 15 gr

WHOLE WHOLE BRUSCHETTE WITH TOMATOES, BASIL AND BUFFALO MOZZARELLA

Preparation time: 15 minutes

Cooking time: 10 minutes

(to toast bread)

Doses: 4 bruschettas

Ingredients:

4 slices of wholemeal bread

200g of cherry tomatoes

10 fresh basil leaves

100g of buffalo mozzarella

Extra virgin olive oil

olive (optional)

Salt and Pepper To Taste

Preparation:

Toast the slices of wholemeal bread. Wash the cherry tomatoes and cut them into small pieces. Chop the fresh basil. Cut the buffalo mozzarella into slices. Arrange the cherry tomatoes, chopped basil and buffalo mozzarella on the toasted bread slices. Drizzle with extra virgin olive oil (optional). Salt and pepper to taste. Serve the bruschetta immediately.

Nutritional values (per serving):

Calories: 350 kcal

Protein: 25 gr

Fat: 20 gr

Carbohydrates: 15 gr

WHOLE BREAD CANAPÉS WITH CHICKPEA HUMMUS AND GRILLED VEGETABLES

Preparation time: 25 minutes

Cooking time: 15 minutes

(for grilling vegetables)

Servings: 2 canapés

Ingredients:

2 slices of wholemeal bread

100g of boiled chickpeas

1/2 aubergine

1/2 red pepper

1 tablespoon lemon juice

1 clove of garlic

1 tablespoon tahini

Salt and Pepper To Taste

Preparation:

Toast the slices of wholemeal bread. Wash the aubergine and pepper. Cut the aubergine into slices and the pepper into strips. Grill the vegetables for 10 minutes, or until soft. In a food processor, blend the boiled chickpeas, grilled vegetables, lemon juice, garlic, tahini, extra virgin olive oil (optional), salt and pepper until creamy. Spread the chickpea hummus on the toasted bread slices. Serve the canapés immediately.

Nutritional values (per serving):

Calories: 400 kcal

Protein: 30 gr

Fat: 25 gr

Carbohydrates: 15 gr

ROLLS OF RAW HAM ROLLS WITH MELON AND FRESH CHEESE

Preparation time: 15 minutes

Cooking time: 0 minutes

Doses: 4 rolls

Ingredients:

4 slices of raw ham

1/4 of a ripe melon

100g of fresh cheese

(like ricotta or robiola)

Fresh basil (optional)

Salt and Pepper To Taste

Preparation:

Cut the melon into thin slices. Spread the fresh cheese on the melon slices. Arrange a slice of raw ham on each slice of melon with fresh cheese. Roll up the melon slices to form rolls. Decorate with fresh basil (optional). Salt and pepper to taste. Serve the rolls immediately.

Nutritional values (per serving):

Calories: 300 kcal

Protein: 20 gr

Fat: 15 gr

Carbohydrates: 15 gr

QUINOA FRITTERS WITH SPINACH AND LIGHT CHEESE

Preparation time: 20 minutes

Cooking time: 10 minutes

Servings: 4 pancakes

Ingredients:

50g of quinoa

100g of spinach

50 g of cheese

light grated

1 egg

1 tablespoon of skimmed milk

1 tablespoon of oil

extra virgin olive oil

Salt and Pepper To Taste

Preparation:

Rinse the quinoa under running water. Cook the quinoa in boiling salted water for 15 minutes. Drain it and cool it. Wash the spinach and boil them in a little boiling water for 2 minutes. Remove the spinach and squeeze it well. In a bowl, mix the quinoa, chopped spinach, grated light cheese, egg, skimmed milk, extra virgin olive oil, salt and pepper. Heat the extra virgin olive oil in a non-stick pan. Pour a spoonful of pancake mixture into the pan and cook for 2-3 minutes per side, or until golden brown. Drain the pancakes on absorbent paper. Serve the pancakes immediately. Nutritional values (per serving): Calories: 250 kcal

Protein: 20 gr

Fat: 10 gr

Carbohydrates: 20 gr

TUNA SALAD WITH CANNELLINI BEANS, RED ONION AND PARSLEY

Preparation time: 20 minutes

Cooking time: 0 minutes

Doses: 1 person

Ingredients:

120g of natural tuna

100g of boiled cannellini beans

1/2 red onion

Fresh parsley

Extra virgin olive oil

olive (optional)

Lemon juice (optional)

Salt and Pepper To Taste

Preparation:

Chop the tuna. Rinse the cannellini beans under running water. Cut the red onion into thin slices. Chop the fresh parsley. In a bowl, mix the tuna, cannellini beans, red onion, fresh parsley, extra virgin olive oil (optional), lemon juice (optional), salt and pepper. Serve the salad immediately.

Nutritional values (per serving):

Calories: 400 kcal

Protein: 35 gr

Fat: 20 gr

Carbohydrates: 25 gr

WHOLE BREAD CROUTTONS WITH CREAM CHEESE AND COOKED HAM

Preparation time: 15 minutes

Cooking time: 0 minutes

Servings: 4 croutons

Ingredients:

4 slices of wholemeal bread

100g of fresh cheese

(like ricotta or robiola)

50 g of cooked ham

Fresh basil (optional)

Extra virgin olive oil

olive (optional)

Salt and Pepper To Taste

Preparation:

Toast the slices of wholemeal bread. In a bowl, mix the fresh cheese, chopped cooked ham, chopped fresh basil (optional), extra virgin olive oil (optional), salt and pepper. Spread the cream cheese and ham on the wholemeal bread croutons. Serve the croutons immediately.

Nutritional values (per serving):

Calories: 250 kcal

Protein: 20 gr

Fat: 15 gr

Carbohydrates: 15 gr

CHICKEN SALAD WITH AVOCADO, CORN AND GREEK YOGURT SAUCE

Preparation time: 25 minutes

Cooking time: 10 minutes

Doses: 1 person

Ingredients:

100g of chicken breast

1/2 ripe avocado

1 tablespoon of corn

100g of Greek yogurt

Lime juice (optional)

Extra virgin olive oil

olive (optional)

Salt and Pepper To Taste

Preparation:

Cook the chicken breast on the grill or in a pan for 10 minutes. Cut the chicken into small pieces. Cut the avocado into small pieces. In a bowl, mix the chicken, avocado, corn, Greek yogurt, lime juice (optional), extra virgin olive oil (optional), salt, and pepper. Serve the salad immediately. You can add other ingredients to the salad, such as olives, tomatoes or herbs.

Nutritional values (per serving):

Calories: 450 kcal

Protein: 40 gr

Fat: 25 gr

Carbohydrates: 10 gr

RECIPES
FIRST DISHES

ATTACK PHASE

KONJAC PENNE WITH GENOVESE PESTO

Preparation time: 10 minutes

Cooking time: 5 minutes

Doses: 1 person

Ingredients:

100g of konjac pens

50 g of Genoese pesto

25 g of cherry tomatoes

Fresh basil (optional)

Salt and Pepper To Taste

Preparation:

Rinse the konjac pens: Rinse the konjac pens under running water to remove any preservative liquid. Cook the konjac penne: Cook the konjac penne in boiling water for 2-3 minutes. Drain the konjac penne: Drain the konjac penne and drain well. Season the konjac penne: In a bowl, season the konjac penne with the Genoese pesto. Add the cherry tomatoes: Cut the cherry tomatoes in half and add them to the seasoned konjac penne.

Decorate with fresh basil (optional): If desired, decorate the dish with fresh basil leaves. Salt and pepper to taste: Salt and pepper to taste. Serve the konjac penne with Genoese pesto immediately, piping hot.

Nutritional values (per serving):

Calories: 125 kcal

Protein: 10 gr

Fat: 7.5 gr

Carbohydrates: 2.5 gr

CAULIFLOWER RISOTTO WITH PORCINI MUSHROOMS

Preparation time: 20 minutes

Cooking time: 15 minutes

Doses: 1 person

Ingredients:

1/4 of cauliflower

50 g of porcini mushrooms

1/2 onion

25 g of grated parmesan

Vegetable broth (optional)

Extra virgin olive oil

Salt and Pepper To Taste

Preparation:

Cut the cauliflower: Cut the cauliflower into florets. Wash the porcini mushrooms: Wash the porcini mushrooms and cut them into slices. Chop the onion: Finely chop the onion. Fry the onion: In a pan, heat the extra virgin olive oil and fry the onion until it becomes transparent. Add the porcini mushrooms: Add the chopped porcini mushrooms to the onion and cook for 2-3 minutes. Add the cauliflower: Add the cauliflower florets to the pan and cook them for about 5 minutes. Add vegetable broth (optional): If necessary, add a little vegetable broth to help cook the cauliflower.

Cook the cauliflower: Cook the cauliflower until soft, about 10 minutes. Stir in the grated parmesan: Remove the pan from the heat and stir in the risotto with the grated parmesan. Salt and pepper to taste: Salt and pepper to taste. Serve immediately: Serve the cauliflower risotto with porcini mushrooms immediately, piping hot.

Nutritional values (per serving):

Calories: 150 kcal

Protein: 12.5 gr

Fat: 7.5 gr

Carbohydrates: 5 gr

COURGETTES LASAGNA WITH TURKEY SAUCE

Preparation time: 40 minutes

Cooking time: 45 minutes

Doses: 1 person

Ingredients

200 g of courgettes

200g of minced turkey

400 g of peeled tomatoes

1 onion

1 clove of garlic

Fresh basil

30 g of parmesan

light grated (optional)

2 tablespoons extra virgin olive oil

Salt and Pepper To Taste

Preparation:

Prepare the ragù (20 minutes): Chop onion and garlic. Saute the onion in olive oil until transparent. Add garlic and cook for 1 minute. Add ground turkey and cook crumbling it for 10 minutes. Add peeled tomatoes, basil, salt and pepper. Cook over low heat for 20 minutes, stirring. Prepare the courgettes (5 minutes): Wash and cut the courgettes into thin slices (3 mm). Assemble the lasagna (10 minutes): Spread a first layer of ragù in a non-stick pan. Cover with the courgette slices. Repeat layers, ending with ragù. Cover the pan with foil.

Bake in a preheated oven at 180°C for 30 minutes. Uncover the pan and sprinkle with parmesan (optional). Bake for a further 15 minutes until golden brown. Serve (10 minutes): Let the lasagna rest for 10 minutes before serving.

Nutritional values (per serving):

Calories: 450 kcal

Protein: 40 gr

Fat: 25 gr

Carbohydrates: 10 gr

CAULIFLOWER OMELETTE WITH TOMATO AND MOZZARELLA

Preparation time: 20 minutes

Cooking time: 20 minutes

Doses: 1 person

Ingredients:

200g of cauliflower

3 eggs

50 g of light mozzarella

100g of cherry tomatoes

Fresh basil

1 tablespoon of oil

extra virgin olive oil

Salt and Pepper To Taste

Preparation:

Prepare the cauliflower (10 minutes): Wash and cut the cauliflower into florets. Steam for 10 minutes until soft. Prepare the omelette (10 minutes): Beat the eggs with salt and pepper in a bowl. Heat the oil in a non-stick pan. Pour the egg mixture into the pan. Distribute evenly. Assemble the omelette (5 minutes): Arrange the cooked cauliflower, halved cherry tomatoes and sliced or grated mozzarella on the omelette. Cooking (15 minutes): Cover the pan with a lid. Cook over low heat for 15 minutes. Check for doneness and cook until golden brown. Serve (5 minutes): Enjoy the omelette hot. Nutritional values (per serving): Calories: 300 kcal

Protein: 25 gr

Fat: 15 gr

Carbohydrates: 10 gr

SCRAMBLED EGGS WITH SALMON AND SPINACH

Preparation time: 10 minutes

Cooking time: 5 minutes

Doses: 1 person

Ingredients:

2 eggs

100g of smoked salmon

100g of fresh spinach

1 tablespoon of oil

extra virgin olive oil

Salt and Pepper To Taste

Preparation:

Fry the oil: Heat the extra virgin olive oil in a non-stick pan.

Cook the spinach: Add the washed spinach and cook for a couple of minutes until wilted. Add the salmon: Add the smoked salmon cut into strips and cook for another minute. Beat the eggs: Beat the eggs in a bowl with a pinch of salt and pepper. Pour in the eggs: Pour the beaten eggs into the pan with the spinach and salmon. Cook the eggs: Cook the scrambled eggs over medium-low heat, stirring occasionally, until the desired consistency is reached. Serve: Serve the scrambled eggs with salmon and spinach immediately. Nutritional values (per serving):

Calories: 250 kcal

Protein: 25 gr

Fat: 15 gr

Carbohydrates: 0 gr

TUNA SALAD WITH TOMATOES AND OLIVES

Preparation time: 10 minutes

Cooking time: 0 minutes

Doses: 1 person

Ingredients:

120g of canned tuna

1 medium tomato

50 g of pitted black olives

1 tablespoon of oil

extra virgin olive oil

Fresh oregano (optional)

Salt and Pepper To Taste

Preparation:

Cut the tomato: Cut the tomato into small pieces. Chop the olives: Chop the black olives. Assemble the salad: In a bowl, combine the drained tuna, tomato, olives, extra virgin olive oil, fresh oregano (optional), salt and pepper. Mix the ingredients: Mix the ingredients well. Serve: Serve the tuna salad with tomatoes and olives chilled.

Nutritional values (per serving):

Calories: 200 kcal

Protein: 20 gr

Fat: 10 gr

Carbohydrates: 5 gr

OMELETTE WITH MUSHROOMS AND CHEESE

Preparation time: 10 minutes

Cooking time: 5 minutes

Doses: 1 person

Ingredients:

2 eggs

50 g of mushrooms

fresh (of your choice)

20 g of cheese

grated light

1 tablespoon butter

Salt and Pepper To Taste

Preparation:

Fry the butter: Fry the butter in a non-stick pan. Cook the mushrooms: Wash and slice the mushrooms. Add them to the pan and cook for about 5 minutes, or until tender. Beat the eggs: Beat the eggs in a bowl with a pinch of salt and pepper. Pour in the eggs: Pour the beaten eggs into the pan with the mushrooms. Sprinkle with cheese: Sprinkle with light grated cheese. Cook the omelette: Cook the omelette over medium-low heat, folding it in half when the edges begin to firm up. Serve the omelette with mushrooms and cheese piping hot.

Nutritional values (per serving):

Calories: 280 kcal

Protein: 22 gr

Fat: 20 gr

Carbohydrates: 2 gr

GRILLED CHICKEN SALAD WITH AVOCADO AND CUCUMBERS

Preparation time: 15 minutes

Cooking time: 10 minutes

Doses: 1 person

Ingredients:

150g of chicken breast

1/2 ripe avocado

1 medium cucumber

1 tablespoon of oil

extra virgin olive oil

Lemon juice (optional)

Salt and Pepper To Taste

Preparation:

Cook the chicken breast on the grill or in a non-stick pan for about 10 minutes per side, or until golden brown and cooked through. Cut the cucumber: Wash the cucumber and cut it into thin slices. Chop the avocado: Chop the ripe avocado into a bowl. Season the avocado: Drizzle the avocado with a drizzle of lemon juice (optional) to prevent it from blackening. Assemble the salad: In a large bowl, combine the sliced grilled chicken, the sliced cucumber, the chopped avocado, the extra virgin olive oil, salt and pepper to taste. Mix the ingredients: Mix the ingredients well to combine everything. Serve the grilled chicken salad with avocado and cucumbers chilled. Nutritional values (per serving):

Calories: 300 kcal, Protein: 30 gr

Fat: 18 g, Carbohydrates: 5 g

BRESAOLA SALAD WITH ARUGULA, PARMESAN AND MELON

Preparation time: 10 minutes

Cooking time: 0 minutes

Doses: 1 person

Ingredients:

100g of bresaola

100g of Arugula

50 g of parmesan

150 g of melon

Extra virgin olive oil

Balsamic vinegar

Salt and Pepper To Taste

Preparation:

Cut the melon into slices and then into cubes. In a serving dish, arrange the Arugula, sliced bresaola, diced melon and flaked parmesan. Drizzle the salad with a drizzle of extra virgin olive oil and balsamic vinegar. Add salt and pepper to taste. Serve the bresaola salad with Arugula, parmesan and melon fresh.

Nutritional values (per serving):

Calories: 350 kcal

Protein: 30 gr

Fat: 15 gr

Carbohydrates: 5 gr

KONJAC SPAGHETTI WITH CLAMS AND TOMATOES

Preparation time: 15 minutes

Cooking time: 10 minutes

Doses: 1 person

Ingredients:

200g of konjac spaghetti

200g of clams

200g of cherry tomatoes

1 clove of garlic

1/2 glass of dry white wine

Fresh parsley

Extra virgin olive oil

Salt and Pepper To Taste

Preparation:

Rinse the clams carefully under running water to remove any impurities. In a pan, heat the extra virgin olive oil and fry the chopped garlic for a minute. Add the clams to the pan and deglaze with the white wine. Cover the pan and cook the clams for about 5 minutes, or until they open. Cut the cherry tomatoes in half and add them to the clams. Cook for another couple of minutes. Rinse and drain the konjac spaghetti. Add the drained konjac to the pan with the clams and cherry tomatoes. Mix well to combine everything. Add chopped fresh parsley, salt and pepper to taste. Serve the konjac spaghetti with clams and cherry tomatoes piping hot. Nutritional values (per serving):

Calories: 250 kcal, Protein: 25 gr

Fat: 10 g, Carbohydrates: 5 g

FENNEL CREAM WITH SHRIMPS

Preparation time: 20 minutes

Cooking time: 30 minutes

Doses: 1 person

Ingredients:

200 g of fennel

1/2 onion

1/2 medium potato

350 ml of vegetable broth

100g of cleaned shrimps

Extra virgin olive oil

Salt and Pepper To Taste

Preparation:

Wash and clean the fennel, onion and potato. Cut the fennel into small pieces, the onion into slices and the potato into cubes. In a pan, heat the extra virgin olive oil and fry the onion for a couple of minutes. Add the fennel and potato and cook for about 5 minutes, stirring occasionally. Pour in the vegetable broth and bring to the boil. Cook for about 20 minutes, or until the fennel and potato are tender. Blend the mixture with a blender until you obtain a smooth cream. Add the shrimp to the cream and cook for another minute. Season with salt and pepper to taste. Serve the fennel cream with prawns piping hot. Nutritional values (per portion): Calories: 175 kcal, Protein: 15 gr

Fat: 7.5 gr

Carbohydrates: 5 gr

LIGHT FISH SOUP WITH MIXED VEGETABLES

Preparation time: 30 minutes

Cooking time: 40 minutes

Doses: 1 person

Ingredients:

250 g of mixed fish (including

cod, sea bream, mackerel)

100 g of mixed vegetables (between

including carrots, courgettes, potatoes)

1/2 onion

1/4 clove of garlic

750 ml of vegetable broth

Extra virgin olive oil

Fresh parsley

Salt and Pepper To Taste

Preparation:

Wash and clean the fish. Cut the vegetables into small pieces. In a pan, heat the extra virgin olive oil and fry the chopped onion and garlic for a couple of minutes. Add the mixed vegetables and cook for about 5 minutes, stirring occasionally. Pour in the vegetable broth and bring to the boil. Cook for about 20 minutes, or until the vegetables are tender. Add the fish and cook for another 10 minutes, or until the fish is cooked through. Season with salt and pepper to taste. Sprinkle with chopped fresh parsley. Serve the light fish soup with mixed vegetables piping hot. Nutritional values (per serving):

Calories: 125 kcal

Protein: 15 gr

Fat: 5 gr

Carbohydrates: 2.5 g

TUNA AND MUSHROOM OMELETTE

Preparation time: 10 minutes

Cooking time: 15 minutes

Doses: 1 person

Ingredients:

2 eggs

70 g of natural tuna

50 g of fresh mixed mushrooms

1/2 small onion

1 tablespoon of oil

extra virgin olive oil

Salt and Pepper To Taste

Fresh parsley

chopped (optional)

Preparation:

Finely chop the onion. Wash and slice the mushrooms. Heat the oil in a non-stick pan. Fry the onion for a few minutes, until it softens. Add the mushrooms and cook for 5-7 minutes, stirring often. Add the drained and crumbled tuna. In a bowl, beat the eggs with a pinch of salt and pepper. Pour the egg mixture into the pan with the tuna and mushrooms. Cook the omelette over low heat for about 5 minutes, until the bottom has thickened. Fold the omelette in half and cook for another 2-3 minutes. and serve hot.

Nutritional values:

Calories: approximately 300 kcal

Protein: approximately 35 g

Fat: approximately 15 g

Carbohydrates: approximately 5 g

LIGHT HERB AND CHEESE OMELETTE

Preparation time: 5 minutes

Cooking time: 10 minutes

Doses: 1 person

Ingredients:

2 eggs

20 g of light ricotta

30 g of grated cheese

light (parmesan, grana padano)

Fresh chives to taste

Salt and Pepper To Taste

Extra virgin olive oil

(to grease the pan)

Preparation:

In a bowl, beat the eggs with a pinch of salt and pepper. Add the ricotta, grated cheese and chopped chives. Mix the mixture well. Heat a drizzle of oil in a non-stick pan. Pour the egg mixture into the pan and cook the omelette over low heat for about 5 minutes, until the bottom has thickened. Fold the omelette in half and cook for another 2-3 minutes. Serve hot. You can vary the vegetables and cheese to your liking. For an even lighter version, you can use just egg whites instead of whole eggs.

Nutritional values:

Calories: approximately 250 kcal

Protein: approximately 25 g

Fat: approximately 12 g

Carbohydrates: approximately 3 g

COURGETTE TAGLIATELLE WITH LENTIL SAUCE

Preparation time: 30 minutes

Cooking time: 40 minutes

Doses: 1 person

Ingredients:

1 large courgette

100 g of dried lentils

1/2 small onion

1 small carrot

1 stalk of celery

1 tablespoon of oil

extra virgin olive oil

1 clove of garlic

1 peeled tomato

1 bay leaf

Salt and Pepper To Taste

Fresh basil

chopped (optional)

Preparation:

Wash the lentils and soak them for at least 2 hours. In the meantime, wash the courgette and cut it into thin strips with a potato peeler or a mandolin, creating "tagliatelle". Finely chop the onion, carrot and celery. Heat the oil in a pan. Fry the onion, carrot and celery for a few minutes, until softened. Add the minced garlic and cook for another minute. Add the rinsed lentils, peeled tomato, bay leaf, salt and pepper.

Cover the pot and cook over low heat for about 30 minutes, stirring occasionally, until the lentils are cooked. While the ragù is cooking, cook the courgette "tagliatelle" in boiling salted water for 2-3 minutes. Drain the courgettes and season them with a drizzle of oil. Serve the courgette "tagliatelle" with the hot lentil ragù, sprinkling with chopped fresh basil (optional).

Nutritional values:

Calories: approximately 400 kcal

Protein: approximately 30 g

Fat: approximately 15 g

Carbohydrates: approximately 10 g

WARM CHICKEN SALAD WITH MUSHROOMS AND SOY

Preparation time: 20 minutes

Cooking time: 15 minutes

Doses: 1 person

Ingredients:

120g sliced chicken breast

100 g of fresh mixed mushrooms

2 tablespoons soy sauce

1 tablespoon of oil

extra virgin olive oil

1/2 small onion

1 clove of garlic

1/2 lemon

Mixed green salad to taste

Sesame seeds (optional)

Preparation:

Wash and slice the mushrooms. Finely chop the onion and garlic. Marinate the chicken with soy sauce, oil, the juice of half a lemon, salt and pepper for at least 15 minutes. Heat the oil in a non-stick pan. Fry the onion and garlic for a few minutes, until softened. Add the mushrooms and cook for 5-7 minutes, stirring often. Add the marinated chicken and cook it for about 5 minutes on each side, until it is golden and cooked inside.

In the meantime, prepare the salad by washing the lettuce and placing it on a plate. Add the cooked mushrooms and chicken. Season with a drizzle of oil and the juice of half a lemon. Sprinkle with sesame seeds (optional) and serve warm.

Nutritional values:

Calories: approximately 350 kcal

Protein: approximately 40 g

Fat: approximately 12 g

Carbohydrates: approximately 5 g

VEGETABLE LASAGNA WITH LIGHT BECHAMEL

Preparation time: 45 minutes

Cooking time: 45 minutes

Doses: 1 person

Ingredients:

2 small aubergines

1 medium courgette

1 red pepper

1 small onion

200 g of light béchamel (prepared

with skimmed milk and wholemeal flour)

50 g of light ricotta

50 g of grated light parmesan

Chopped fresh basil (optional)

Salt and Pepper To Taste

Extra virgin olive oil

(to grease the pan)

Preparation:

Wash the aubergines, courgette and pepper. Cut the aubergines into thin slices lengthwise. Grill the aubergines on both sides for a few minutes, until they are slightly wilted. Cut the courgette and pepper into thin slices. Finely chop the onion. Heat a drizzle of oil in a non-stick pan. Fry the onion for a few minutes, until it softens. Add the courgettes and pepper and cook for 5-7 minutes, stirring often. In a bowl, mix the light ricotta with the grated parmesan and a pinch of salt and pepper. Prepare the light béchamel following the instructions on the package. Grease a baking tray with oil.

Arrange a layer of grilled aubergines on the bottom of the pan. Spread a little light béchamel on the aubergines. Spread the layer of cooked vegetables (courgettes and peppers). Add a spoonful of the ricotta and parmesan mixture. Repeat the layers until you run out of ingredients. Finish with a layer of light béchamel. Cook in a preheated oven at 180°C for about 30 minutes, until the lasagna is golden and the béchamel sauce is gratinated. Remove from the oven and let rest for a few minutes before serving.

Nutritional values:

Calories: approximately 450 kcal

Protein: approximately 35 g

Fat: approximately 20 g

Carbohydrates: approximately 15 g

CAULIFLOWER AND PRAWNS RISOTTO

Preparation time: 25 minutes

Cooking time: 20 minutes

Doses: 1 person

Ingredients:

150 g of cauliflower

100 g of cleaned shrimps

1/2 small onion

1 clove of garlic

1/2 glass of dry white wine

400 ml of light vegetable broth

1 tablespoon extra virgin olive oil

Chopped fresh parsley

Salt and Pepper To Taste

Preparation:

Wash the cauliflower and cut it into florets. Finely chop the onion and garlic. Fry the onion and garlic in a non-stick pan with oil for a few minutes, until soft. Add the cauliflower florets and cook for 5 minutes, stirring often. Pour in the white wine and let the alcohol evaporate. Add the hot vegetable broth and cook for about 15 minutes, stirring occasionally, until the cauliflower is soft. In the meantime, cook the prawns in another non-stick pan with a drizzle of oil for a couple of minutes on each side, until they are golden.

Add the cooked shrimp to the risotto and mix gently. Season with salt and pepper to taste. Turn off the heat and stir in the risotto with a spoonful of butter (optional). Serve the risotto hot, sprinkled with fresh chopped parsley.

Nutritional values:

Calories: approximately 450 kcal

Protein: approximately 40 g

Fat: approximately 15 g

Carbohydrates: approximately 30 g

PUMPKIN GNOCCHI WITH SOY RAGU

Preparation time: 40 minutes

Cooking time: 30 minutes

Doses: 1 person

Ingredients:

200 g of pumpkin

50 g of wholemeal flour

1 egg

1 tablespoon grated parmesan

Salt and Pepper To Taste

Extra virgin olive oil

(to grease the pan)

For the soy sauce:

100 g of tofu

1/2 small onion

1 clove of garlic

2 tablespoons soy sauce

1 tablespoon extra virgin olive oil

1 peeled tomato

1/2 glass of light vegetable broth

Salt and Pepper To Taste

Preparation:

Wash the pumpkin and cut it into pieces. Cook the pumpkin by steaming or boiling water for about 15 minutes, until it is soft. Mash the pumpkin with a fork to obtain a puree. Add the wholemeal flour, egg, grated parmesan, salt and pepper. Knead the mixture well until you obtain a smooth and soft dough. If necessary, add a little wholemeal flour or water to adjust the consistency. Form gnocchi with wet hands. Arrange the gnocchi on a floured tray.

For the soy sauce: Crumble the tofu with your hands. Finely chop the onion and garlic. Heat the oil in a non-stick pan. Fry the onion and garlic for a few minutes, until softened. Add the crumbled tofu and cook for 5 minutes, stirring often. Add the soy sauce, peeled tomato, vegetable broth, salt and pepper. Cook the soy sauce for about 15 minutes, stirring occasionally, until it is thick. Add chopped fresh basil (optional). Cooking: Cook the gnocchi in boiling salted water for 2-3 minutes, until they float to the surface. Drain the gnocchi and season them with the hot soy sauce. Nutritional values:

Calories: approximately 400 kcal

Protein: approximately 35 g

Fat: approximately 15 g

Carbohydrates: approximately 20 g

WHOLE WHOLE PASTA WITH CHICKEN AND MUSHROOMS

Preparation time: 25 minutes

Cooking time: 20 minutes

Doses: 1 person

Ingredients:

80 g of wholemeal pasta

120g sliced chicken breast

100 g of fresh mixed mushrooms

1/2 small onion

1 clove of garlic

1 tablespoon of oil

extra virgin olive oil

1/2 glass of wine

dry white (optional)

Chopped fresh parsley

Salt and Pepper To Taste

Preparation:

Wash and slice the mushrooms. Finely chop the onion and garlic. Marinate the chicken with a pinch of salt and pepper for a few minutes. Heat the oil in a non-stick pan. Fry the onion and garlic for a few minutes, until softened. Add the mushrooms and cook for 5-7 minutes, stirring often. Add the marinated chicken and cook it for about 5 minutes on each side, until it is golden and cooked inside. Deglaze with dry white wine (optional) and let the alcohol evaporate.

Cook the wholemeal pasta in boiling salted water for the time indicated on the package. Drain the pasta and season it with a drizzle of oil to prevent it from sticking. Add the pasta to the chicken and mushrooms in the pan and mix well. Season with salt and pepper to taste. Serve the pasta hot, sprinkled with chopped fresh parsley.

Nutritional values:

Calories: approximately 400 kcal

Protein: approximately 35 g

Fat: approximately 15 g

Carbohydrates: approximately 25 g

FISH SOUP WITH
PEARL BARLEY

Preparation time: 30 minutes

Cooking time: 40 minutes

Doses: 1 person

Ingredients:

200 g of fresh mixed fish

(cod, sea bream, sea bass)

50 g of pearl barley

1/2 small onion

1 small carrot

1 stalk of celery

1 clove of garlic

1 peeled tomato

1 liter of vegetable broth

1 tablespoon extra virgin olive oil

Chopped fresh parsley

Salt and Pepper To Taste

Preparation:

Wash the fish and cut it into pieces. Wash the pearl barley and soak it for at least 30 minutes. Finely chop the onion, carrot and celery. Fry the onion, carrot and celery in a pan with oil for a few minutes, until soft. Add the minced garlic and cook for another minute. Add the peeled tomato and mash it with a spoon. Add the vegetable broth and bring to the boil.

Add the drained pearl barley and cook for about 20 minutes, until soft. Add the fish and cook for another 10 minutes, until cooked through. Season with salt and pepper to taste. Serve the soup hot, sprinkled with chopped fresh parsley.

Nutritional values:

Calories: approximately 350 kcal

Protein: approximately 30 g

Fat: approximately 10 g

Carbohydrates: approximately 20 g

WHOLE WHOLE CANNELLONI WITH RICOTTA AND BEETS

Preparation time: 40 minutes

Cooking time: 30 minutes

Doses: 1 person

Ingredients:

4 wholemeal cannelloni

200 g of ricotta

150 g of chard

1/2 small onion

1 clove of garlic

1 tablespoon grated parmesan

1 tablespoon extra virgin olive oil

Light béchamel (prepared with milk skimmed and wholemeal flour)

Chopped fresh parsley

Salt and Pepper To Taste

Preparation:

Wash the beets and boil them in boiling salted water for a few minutes. Drain them and squeeze them well. Finely chop the onion and garlic. Fry the onion and garlic in a pan with oil for a few minutes, until soft. Add the chopped beets and cook for 5 minutes, stirring often. In a bowl, mix the ricotta with the grated parmesan, a pinch of salt and pepper. Add the cooked beets and mix well. Cook the wholemeal cannelloni in boiling salted water for the time indicated on the package.

Drain them and fill them with the ricotta and chard mixture. Arrange the cannelloni on a baking tray. Cover the cannelloni with the light béchamel. Cook in a preheated oven at 180°C for about 20 minutes, until the béchamel sauce is gratinated. Remove from the oven and let rest for a few minutes before serving. Sprinkle with chopped fresh parsley.

Nutritional values:

Calories: approximately 400 kcal

Protein: approximately 35 g

Fat: approximately 15 g

Carbohydrates: approximately 25 g

WHOLEWHEAT PIE WITH SEASONAL VEGETABLES

Preparation time: 45 minutes

Cooking time: 40 minutes

Doses: 1 person

Ingredients:

1 roll of wholemeal puff pastry

200 g of seasonal vegetables

(courgettes, peppers, aubergines)

1/2 small onion

1 clove of garlic

1 tablespoon of oil

extra virgin olive oil

2 eggs

50 g of ricotta

50 g of grated parmesan

Chopped fresh parsley

Salt and Pepper To Taste

Preparation:

Wash seasonal vegetables and cut them into small pieces. Finely chop the onion and garlic. Fry the onion and garlic in a pan with oil for a few minutes, until soft. Add the seasonal vegetables and cook them for 10-15 minutes, stirring often. In a bowl, beat the eggs with the ricotta, the grated parmesan, a pinch of salt and pepper. Add the cooked vegetables to the egg and ricotta mixture and mix well. Unroll the wholemeal puff pastry and line a baking tray.

Pour the vegetable and ricotta mixture onto the puff pastry. Bake in a preheated oven at 180°C for about 40 minutes, until the savory pie is golden. Remove from the oven and let rest for a few minutes before serving. Sprinkle with chopped fresh parsley.

Nutritional values:

Calories: approximately 450 kcal

Protein: approximately 30 g

Fat: approximately 20 g

Carbohydrates: approximately 30 g

**WHOLE WHOLE PASTA
AND LEGUMES SOUP**

Preparation time: 30 minutes

Cooking time: 40 minutes

Doses: 1 person

Ingredients:

50 g of wholemeal pasta

100 g of mixed legumes

(e.g. chickpeas, lentils, beans)

1/2 small onion

1 small carrot, 1 celery stalk

1 clove of garlic, 1 peeled tomato

1 liter of vegetable broth

1 tablespoon extra virgin olive oil

Chopped fresh parsley

Salt and Pepper To Taste

Preparation:

Rinse the mixed legumes and soak them for at least 30 minutes. Finely chop the onion, carrot and celery. Fry the onion, carrot and celery in a pan with oil for a few minutes, until soft. Add the minced garlic and cook for another minute. Add the peeled tomato and mash it with a spoon. Add the vegetable broth and bring to the boil. Add the drained legumes and cook for about 20 minutes, until they are tender. Add the wholemeal pasta and cook for the time indicated on the package. Season with salt and pepper to taste. Serve the soup hot, sprinkled with fresh chopped parsley. Nutritional values: Calories: approximately 350 kcal

Protein: approximately 30 g, Fat: approximately 10 g

Carbohydrates: approximately 25 g

WHOLE WHOLE PASTA WITH TOMATO AND BASIL

Preparation time: 20 minutes

Cooking time: 20 minutes

Doses: 1 person

Ingredients:

80 g of wholemeal pasta

400 g of peeled tomatoes

1/2 small onion

1 clove of garlic

1 tablespoon extra virgin olive oil

Chopped fresh basil

Salt and Pepper To Taste

Preparation:

Wash the peeled tomatoes and cut them into small pieces. Finely chop the onion and garlic. Fry the onion and garlic in a pan with oil for a few minutes, until soft. Add the peeled tomatoes, a pinch of salt and pepper. Cook for about 15 minutes, stirring occasionally, until the sauce is thick. Cook the wholemeal pasta in boiling salted water for the time indicated on the package. Drain the pasta and season it with the tomato sauce. Add the chopped fresh basil and mix well. Serve the pasta hot.

Nutritional values:

Calories: approximately 350 kcal

Protein: approximately 25 g

Fat: approximately 10 g

Carbohydrates: approximately 30 g

RISOTTO WITH MIXED MUSHROOMS

Preparation time: 25 minutes

Cooking time: 20 minutes

Doses: 1 person

Ingredients:

80 g of Carnaroli rice

100 g of fresh mixed mushrooms

1/2 small onion

1 clove of garlic

1 tablespoon extra virgin olive oil

1/2 glass of dry white wine (optional)

400 ml of light vegetable broth

Chopped fresh parsley

Salt and Pepper To Taste

Preparation:

Wash and slice the mushrooms. Finely chop the onion and garlic. Fry the onion and garlic in a non-stick pan with oil for a few minutes, until soft. Add the mushrooms and cook for 5-7 minutes, stirring often. Deglaze with dry white wine (optional) and let the alcohol evaporate. Add the Carnaroli rice and toast for a minute. Add the hot vegetable broth one ladle at a time, stirring constantly, and cook for about 15 minutes, until the rice is creamy. Season with salt and pepper to taste. Turn off the heat and stir in the risotto with a spoonful of butter (optional). Serve the risotto hot, sprinkled with fresh chopped parsley. Nutritional values:

Calories: approximately 400 kcal, Proteins: approximately 30 g

Fat: approximately 15 g, Carbohydrates: approximately 25 g

MIXED LEGUME SOUP

Preparation time: 40 minutes

Cooking time: 40 minutes

Doses: 1 person

Ingredients:

100 g of mixed legumes

(chickpeas, lentils, beans)

1/2 small onion

1 small carrot

1 stalk of celery

1 clove of garlic

1 peeled tomato

1 liter of vegetable broth

1 tablespoon extra virgin olive oil

Chopped fresh parsley

Salt and Pepper To Taste

Preparation:

Rinse the mixed legumes and soak them for at least 30 minutes. Finely chop the onion, carrot and celery. Fry the onion, carrot and celery in a pan with oil for a few minutes, until soft. Add the minced garlic and cook for another minute. Add the peeled tomato and mash it with a spoon. Add the vegetable broth and bring to the boil. Add the drained legumes and cook for about 20 minutes, until they are tender. Season with salt and pepper to taste. Serve the soup hot, sprinkled with chopped fresh parsley.

Nutritional values:

Calories: approximately 350 kcal

Protein: approximately 30 g

Fat: approximately 10 g

Carbohydrates: approximately 25 g

WHOLEWHEAT PENNE WITH AUBERGINES DRIED TOMATOES AND BASIL

Preparation time: 30 minutes

Cooking time: 30 minutes

Doses: 1 person

Ingredients:

80 g of wholemeal penne

1 small aubergine

5 dried tomatoes

1/2 small onion

1 clove of garlic

1 tablespoon extra virgin olive oil

Chopped fresh basil

Salt and Pepper To Taste

Preparation:

Wash the aubergine and cut it into cubes. Hydrate the dried tomatoes in warm water for 10 minutes. Finely chop the onion and garlic. Fry the onion and garlic in a pan with oil for a few minutes, until soft. Add the diced aubergine and cook for 10 minutes, stirring often. Add the dried tomatoes, squeezed and cut into pieces. Cook for another 5 minutes, stirring gently. Cook the wholemeal penne in boiling salted water for the time indicated on the package. Drain the pasta and season it with the aubergine and dried tomato sauce. Add the chopped fresh basil and mix well. Serve the penne hot.

Nutritional values:

Calories: approximately 400 kcal, Protein: approximately 25 g

Fat: approximately 15 g, Carbohydrates: approximately 30 g

RICOTTA AND SPINACH GNOCCHI

Preparation time: 30 minutes

Cooking time: 20 minutes

Doses: 1 person

Ingredients:

200 g of ricotta

100 g of spinach

50 g of wholemeal flour

1 egg

1 pinch of nutmeg

Salt and Pepper To Taste

Preparation:

Wash the spinach and boil them in boiling salted water for a minute. Drain them and squeeze them well. In a bowl, mix the ricotta, egg, wholemeal flour, a pinch of nutmeg, salt and pepper. Add the chopped spinach and mix well. Form gnocchi with the mixture obtained. Cook the gnocchi in boiling salted water for a couple of minutes, until they float to the surface. Drain the gnocchi and season them with a drizzle of oil and a pinch of grated parmesan (optional).

Nutritional values:

Calories: approximately 400 kcal

Protein: approximately 35 g

Fat: approximately 15 g

Carbohydrates: approximately 20 g

PENNE WITH GRILLED VEGETABLES AND FETA

Preparation time: 20 minutes

Cooking time: 20 minutes

Doses: 1 person

Ingredients:

80 g of wholemeal Penne

1 small courgette

1 small pepper

1 small aubergine

100 g of feta

1 tablespoon extra virgin olive oil

Chopped fresh basil

Salt and Pepper To Taste

Preparation:

Wash the vegetables and cut them into strips. Grill the vegetables for about 10 minutes, turning them often. Cook the wholemeal penne in boiling salted water for the time indicated on the package. Melt the feta in a pan with a drizzle of oil for a minute. Drain the pasta and season it with the grilled vegetables and melted feta. Add the chopped fresh basil and mix well. Serve the penne hot.

Nutritional values:

Calories: approximately 450 kcal

Protein: approximately 30 g

Fat: approximately 20 g

Carbohydrates: approximately 25 g

WHOLE WHOLE RISOTTO WITH COURGETTES AND PRAWNS

Preparation time: 25 minutes

Cooking time: 20 minutes

Doses: 1 person

Ingredients:

80 g of wholemeal Carnaroli rice

100 g of courgettes

100 g of cleaned Prawns

1/2 small onion

1 clove of garlic

1 tablespoon extra virgin olive oil

1/2 glass of dry white wine (optional)

400 ml of light vegetable broth

Chopped fresh parsley

Salt and Pepper To Taste

Preparation:

Wash the courgettes and cut them into cubes. Shell the prawns and clean them. Finely chop the onion and garlic. Fry the onion and garlic in a non-stick pan with oil for a few minutes, until soft. Add the diced courgettes and cook for 5-7 minutes, stirring often. Deglaze with dry white wine (optional) and let the alcohol evaporate. Add the wholemeal Carnaroli rice and toast for a minute. Add the hot vegetable broth one ladle at a time, stirring constantly, and cook for about 15 minutes, until the rice is creamy.

Add the Prawns and cook for another 2-3 minutes. Season with salt and pepper to taste. Turn off the heat and stir in the risotto with a spoonful of butter (optional). Serve the risotto hot, sprinkled with fresh chopped parsley.

Nutritional values:

Calories: approximately 500 kcal

Protein: approximately 40 g

Fat: approximately 20 g

Carbohydrates: approximately 30 g

WHOLE WHOLE TORTELLINI WITH TURKEY SAUCE

Preparation time: 45 minutes

Cooking time: 40 minutes

Doses: 1 person

Ingredients:

200 g of wholemeal tortellini

200 g of minced turkey

1/2 small onion

1 small carrot

1 stalk of celery

1 clove of garlic

400 g of peeled tomatoes

1 tablespoon extra virgin olive oil

Chopped fresh basil

Salt and Pepper To Taste

Preparation:

Finely chop the onion, carrot and celery. Fry the onion, carrot and celery in a pan with oil for a few minutes, until soft. Add the minced garlic and cook for another minute. Add the ground turkey and cook for about 5 minutes, stirring often. Add the peeled tomatoes, a pinch of salt and pepper. Cook for about 20 minutes, stirring occasionally, until the ragù is thick. Cook the wholemeal tortellini in boiling salted water for the time indicated on the package. Drain the tortellini and season them with the turkey ragù. Add the chopped fresh basil and mix well. Serve the tortellini hot. Nutritional values:

Calories: approximately 600 kcal, Proteins: approximately 50 g

Fat: approximately 25 g, Carbohydrates: approximately 40 g

RECIPES
SECOND DISHES

SALMON FILLET WITH LEMON WITH GRILLED VEGETABLES

Preparation time: 20 minutes

Cooking time: 20 minutes

Doses: 1 person

Ingredients:

150 g of salmon fillet

1 lemon

1 tablespoon extra virgin olive oil

Chopped fresh parsley

Salt and Pepper To Taste

Grilled vegetables to taste

(courgettes, peppers, aubergines)

Preparation:

Wash the salmon fillet and dry it well with kitchen paper. Salt and pepper the salmon on both sides. Squeeze the juice of a lemon onto the salmon and massage gently. Heat the extra virgin olive oil in a non-stick pan. Cook the salmon fillet for about 5 minutes per side, until golden and cooked through. Meanwhile, grill vegetables to taste. Serve the salmon fillet with the grilled vegetables and garnish with chopped fresh parsley.

Nutritional values:

Calories: approximately 450 kcal

Protein: approximately 40 g

Fat: approximately 20 g

Carbohydrates: approximately 5 g

BAKED CHICKEN BREAST WITH AROMATIC HERBS

Preparation time: 20 minutes

Cooking time: 30 minutes

Doses: 1 person

Ingredients:

150 g of chicken breast

1 tablespoon of oil

extra virgin olive oil

1 clove of garlic

Fresh rosemary

Fresh sage

Fresh thyme

Salt and Pepper To Taste

Preparation:

Preheat the oven to 180°C. Wash the chicken breast and dry it well with kitchen paper. In a bowl, mix the extra virgin olive oil, minced garlic, fresh rosemary, fresh sage and fresh thyme. Salt and pepper the chicken breast on both sides. Baste the chicken breast with the herb mixture. Cook the chicken breast in the oven for about 30 minutes, until golden and cooked through. Serve the chicken breast with a side of vegetables of your choice.

Nutritional values:

Calories: approximately 350 kcal

Protein: approximately 45 g

Fat: approximately 15 g

Carbohydrates: approximately 0 g

ASPARAGUS AND MUSHROOM OMELETTE

Preparation time: 15 minutes

Cooking time: 10 minutes

Doses: 1 person

Ingredients:

2 eggs

100 g of asparagus

50 g of mixed mushrooms

1/2 small onion

1 tablespoon of oil

extra virgin olive oil

Chopped fresh parsley

Salt and Pepper To Taste

Preparation:

Wash the asparagus and cut them into small pieces. Wash the mushrooms and cut them into slices. Finely chop the onion. Fry the onion in a non-stick pan with oil for a few minutes, until it softens. Add the asparagus and mushrooms and cook for 5 minutes, stirring often. In a bowl, beat the eggs with a pinch of salt and pepper. Pour the egg mixture into the pan with the asparagus and mushrooms. Cook the omelette for about 5 minutes, until cooked through. Fold the omelette in half and serve. Garnish with chopped fresh parsley.

Nutritional values:

Calories: approximately 300 kcal

Protein: approximately 30 g

Fat: approximately 15 g

Carbohydrates: approximately 5 g

STEAMED SALMON WITH LEMON SAUCE AND HERB

Preparation time: 15 minutes

Cooking time: 10 minutes

Doses: 1 person

Ingredients:

150 g of salmon fillet

1 lemon

1 tablespoon of oil

extra virgin olive oil

Chopped fresh parsley

Chopped fresh dill

Salt and Pepper To Taste

Preparation:

Wash the salmon fillet and dry it well with kitchen paper. Salt and pepper the salmon on both sides. Steam the salmon for about 10 minutes, until cooked. Meanwhile, prepare the lemon and herb sauce: in a bowl, mix the juice of one lemon, the extra virgin olive oil, the chopped fresh parsley and the chopped fresh dill. Serve the steamed salmon with the lemon and herb sauce.

Nutritional values:

Calories: approximately 350 kcal

Protein: approximately 40 g

Fat: approximately 15 g

Carbohydrates: approximately 0 g

GRILLED BEEF FILLET WITH ROASTED TOMATOES

Preparation time: 20 minutes

Cooking time: 20 minutes

Doses: 1 person

Ingredients:

150 g of beef fillet

2 tomatoes

1 tablespoon of oil

extra virgin olive oil

Fresh rosemary

Fresh sage

Salt and Pepper To Taste

Preparation:

Wash the beef fillet and dry it well with kitchen paper. Salt and pepper the beef fillet on both sides. Wash the tomatoes and cut them in half. In a bowl, mix the extra virgin olive oil, fresh rosemary and fresh sage. Brush the tomatoes with the herb mixture. Cook the grilled beef fillet for about 5 minutes on each side, until golden and cooked through. Meanwhile, cook the tomatoes in the oven at 180°C for about 15 minutes, until they are roasted. Serve the beef tenderloin with the roasted tomatoes.

Nutritional values:

Calories: approximately 400 kcal

Protein: approximately 45 g

Fat: approximately 20 g

Carbohydrates: approximately 5 g

GRILLED SWORDFISH WITH SPINACH SIDE SIDE

Preparation time: 20 minutes

Cooking time: 15 minutes

Doses: 1 person

Ingredients:

150 g of swordfish

200 g of spinach

1 clove of garlic

1 tablespoon of oil

extra virgin olive oil

Salt and Pepper To Taste

Preparation:

Wash the swordfish and dry it well with kitchen paper. Salt and pepper the swordfish on both sides. Grill the swordfish for about 5 minutes per side, until golden and cooked through. In the meantime, wash the spinach and boil them in boiling salted water for a minute. Drain them and squeeze them well. In a pan, heat the extra virgin olive oil and fry the chopped garlic for a minute. Add the spinach and cook for 5 minutes, stirring often. Serve the swordfish with the sautéed spinach.

Nutritional values:

Calories: approximately 350 kcal

Protein: approximately 40 g

Fat: approximately 15 g

Carbohydrates: approximately 5 g

TUNA SALAD WITH TOMATOES AND CUCUMBERS

Preparation time: 10 minutes

Cooking time: 0

Doses: 1 person

Ingredients:

150g canned tuna

100 g of cherry tomatoes

1 cucumber

1/2 red onion

1 tablespoon of oil

extra virgin olive oil

Chopped fresh parsley

Salt and Pepper To Taste

Preparation:

Wash the cherry tomatoes and cut them in half. Wash the cucumber and cut it into thin slices. Finely chop the red onion. In a bowl, mix the tuna, cherry tomatoes, cucumber, red onion, extra virgin olive oil, chopped fresh parsley, salt and pepper to taste. Serve the fresh tuna salad.

Nutritional values:

Calories: approximately 350 kcal

Protein: approximately 40 g

Fat: approximately 20 g

Carbohydrates: approximately 5 g

BAKED COD FILLET
WITH TOMATOES
AND OREGANO

Preparation time: 15 minutes

Cooking time: 20 minutes

Doses: 1 person

Ingredients:

150 g of cod fillet

100 g of cherry tomatoes

1 tablespoon of oil

extra virgin olive oil

Fresh oregano

Salt and Pepper To Taste

Preparation:

Preheat the oven to 180°C. Wash the cod fillet and dry it well with kitchen paper. Salt and pepper the cod fillet on both sides. In a baking pan, grease the bottom with extra virgin olive oil. Arrange the cod fillet in the pan and distribute the cherry tomatoes cut in half. Sprinkle with fresh oregano. Bake in the oven for about 20 minutes, until the cod is cooked. Serve the baked cod fillet with cherry tomatoes and oregano.

Nutritional values:

Calories: approximately 300 kcal

Protein: approximately 45 g

Fat: approximately 10 g

Carbohydrates: approximately 5 g

CHICKEN CURRY WITH GRILLED VEGETABLES

Preparation time: 25 minutes

Cooking time: 20 minutes

Doses: 1 person

Ingredients:

150 g of chicken breast

1 tablespoon extra virgin olive oil

1 small onion

1 clove of garlic

1 teaspoon curry powder

400ml coconut milk

100 g of grilled vegetables to taste

(courgettes, peppers, aubergines)

Chopped fresh parsley, Salt and pepper to taste

Preparation:

Wash the chicken breast and dry it well with kitchen paper. Cut the chicken breast into cubes. In a non-stick pan, heat the extra virgin olive oil and fry the chopped onion and chopped garlic for a few minutes, until soft. Add the curry powder and mix well. Add the diced chicken breast and cook for 5 minutes, stirring often. Pour in the coconut milk and cook for about 15 minutes, until the chicken is cooked and the sauce has thickened. Add grilled vegetables to taste and mix gently. Serve the chicken curry with chopped fresh parsley.

Nutritional values:

Calories: approximately 500 kcal, Proteins: approximately 45 g

Fat: approximately 25 g, Carbohydrates: approximately 5 g

GRILLED SALMON WITH CITRUS SAUCE

Preparation time: 15 minutes

Cooking time: 15 minutes

Doses: 1 person

Ingredients:

150 g of salmon fillet

1 lemon

1 orange

1 tablespoon of oil

extra virgin olive oil

Chopped fresh parsley

Salt and Pepper To Taste

Preparation:

Wash the salmon fillet and dry it well with kitchen paper. Salt and pepper the salmon on both sides. Grill the salmon for about 10 minutes per side, until golden and cooked through. In the meantime, prepare the citrus sauce: in a bowl, mix the juice of a lemon, the juice of an orange, the extra virgin olive oil and the chopped fresh parsley. Serve the grilled salmon with the citrus sauce.

Nutritional values:

Calories: approximately 400 kcal

Protein: approximately 40 g

Fat: approximately 20 g

Carbohydrates: approximately 5 g

BEEF STEAK WITH PEPPERS AND ONIONS

Preparation time: 20 minutes

Cooking time: 20 minutes

Doses: 1 person

Ingredients:

150 g of beef steak

1 green pepper

1 small onion

1 tablespoon of oil

extra virgin olive oil

Fresh rosemary

Fresh sage

Salt and Pepper To Taste

Preparation:

Wash the beef steak and dry it well with kitchen paper. Salt and pepper the steak on both sides. Wash the green pepper and cut it into slices. Finely chop the onion. In a non-stick pan, heat the extra virgin olive oil and fry the onion for a few minutes, until it softens. Add the sliced pepper and cook for 5 minutes, stirring often. Grill the steak for about 5 minutes per side, until browned and cooked through. Serve steak with sautéed peppers and onion, garnished with fresh rosemary and fresh sage. Nutritional values:

Calories: approximately 450 kcal

Protein: approximately 50 g

Fat: approximately 20 g

Carbohydrates: approximately 5 g

CHICKEN BREAST STUFFED WITH SPINACH AND SKINNY CHEESE

Preparation time: 25 minutes

Cooking time: 30 minutes

Doses: 1 person

Ingredients:

150 g of chicken breast

200 g of spinach

50 g of ricotta

1 clove of garlic

1 tablespoon of oil

extra virgin olive oil

Fresh sage

Salt and Pepper To Taste

Preparation:

Wash the chicken breast and dry it well with kitchen paper. Open a pocket in the chicken breast with a sharp knife. In a pan, heat the extra virgin olive oil and fry the chopped garlic for a minute. Add the spinach and cook for 5 minutes, stirring often. Drain them and squeeze them well. In a bowl, mix the spinach, ricotta, fresh sage, salt and pepper to taste. Stuff the chicken breast with the spinach and ricotta mixture. Close the chicken breast pocket with cooking string. Cook the chicken breast in the oven at 180°C for about 30 minutes, until golden and cooked. Nutritional values:

Calories: approximately 400 kcal

Protein: approximately 50 g

Fat: approximately 15 g

Carbohydrates: approximately 5 g

GRILLED TUNA WITH TOMATO AND BASIL SAUCE

Preparation time: 15 minutes

Cooking time: 10 minutes

Doses: 1 person

Ingredients:

150 g of fresh tuna

200 g of peeled tomatoes

1/2 small onion

1 clove of garlic

1 tablespoon of oil

extra virgin olive oil

Fresh basil

Salt and Pepper To Taste

Preparation:

Wash the fresh tuna and dry it well with kitchen paper. Salt and pepper the tuna on both sides. Grill the tuna for about 5 minutes on each side, until golden and cooked. In the meantime, prepare the tomato and basil sauce: in a pan, heat the extra virgin olive oil and fry the chopped onion and minced garlic for a few minutes, until they soften. Add the peeled tomatoes and mash them with a fork. Cook for about 10 minutes, stirring often, until the sauce has thickened. Add chopped fresh basil, salt and pepper to taste. Serve the grilled tuna with the tomato and basil sauce. Nutritional values:

Calories: approximately 400 kcal

Protein: approximately 50 g

Fat: approximately 15 g

Carbohydrates: approximately 5 g

COD BAKED IN PAPER WITH MIXED VEGETABLES

Preparation time: 20 minutes

Cooking time: 20 minutes

Doses: 1 person

Ingredients:

150 g of cod fillet

200 g of mixed vegetables

(courgettes, peppers, carrots)

1/2 small onion

1 clove of garlic

1 tablespoon of oil

extra virgin olive oil

Chopped fresh parsley

Salt and Pepper To Taste

Preparation:

Preheat the oven to 180°C. Wash the cod fillet and dry it well with kitchen paper. Wash the mixed vegetables and cut them into pieces. In a bowl, mix the vegetables with the extra virgin olive oil, salt and pepper to taste. Place the cod fillet on a sheet of baking paper. Distribute the vegetables around the cod. Close the baking paper bag. Bake in the oven for about 20 minutes, until the cod is cooked and the vegetables are soft. Serve the cod in foil with chopped fresh parsley.

Nutritional values:

Calories: approximately 350 kcal

Protein: approximately 45 g

Fat: approximately 10 g

Carbohydrates: approximately 5 g

BAKED TURKEY WITH MEDITERRANEAN SPICES

Preparation time: 25 minutes

Cooking time: 40 minutes

Doses: 1 person

Ingredients:

150g turkey breast

1 tablespoon of oil

extra virgin olive oil

1 teaspoon dried oregano

1/2 teaspoon dried thyme

1/4 teaspoon sweet paprika

Salt and Pepper To Taste

Preparation:

Preheat the oven to 180°C. Wash the turkey breast and dry it well with kitchen paper. In a bowl, mix the extra virgin olive oil, dried oregano, dried thyme, sweet paprika, salt and pepper to taste. Sprinkle the spice mixture over the turkey breast. Place the turkey breast on a baking tray lined with baking paper. Bake in the oven for about 40 minutes, until the turkey is browned and cooked through.

Nutritional values:

Calories: approximately 350 kcal

Protein: approximately 50 g

Fat: approximately 15 g

Carbohydrates: approximately 0 g

VEAL MILANESE WITH MIXED SALAD

Preparation time: 20 minutes

Cooking time: 15 minutes

Doses: 1 person

Ingredients:

150 g of veal slice

1 egg

Durum wheat gluten flour

Bread crumbs

Seed oil for frying

Mixed salad

(lettuce, cherry tomatoes, cucumbers)

Lemon

Extra virgin olive oil

Salt and Pepper To Taste

Preparation:

Beat the egg in a shallow dish. Place the durum wheat gluten flour in another shallow dish. Mix the breadcrumbs with a pinch of salt in a third shallow dish. Dip the veal slice in the durum wheat gluten flour, then in the beaten egg and finally in the breadcrumbs. Heat the vegetable oil in a non-stick pan. Fry the veal slice for about 5 minutes on each side, until golden and cooked. In the meantime, prepare the mixed salad: wash and dry the lettuce, cut the cherry tomatoes and cucumbers. Season the salad with lemon juice, extra virgin olive oil, salt and pepper to taste. Serve the Milanese cutlet with the mixed salad. Nutritional values:

Calories: approximately 500 kcal

Protein: approximately 50 g

Fat: approximately 30 g

Carbohydrates: approximately 5 g

BAKED SALMON TROUT WITH POTATOES

Preparation time: 20 minutes

Cooking time: 30 minutes

Doses: 1 person

Ingredients:

150 g of salmon trout

200 g of potatoes

1 tablespoon of oil

extra virgin olive oil

Fresh rosemary

Fresh sage

Salt and Pepper To Taste

Preparation:

Preheat the oven to 180°C. Wash the salmon trout and dry it well with kitchen paper. Salt and pepper the salmon trout on both sides. Peel the potatoes and cut them into slices. Place the sliced potatoes on a baking tray and season them with extra virgin olive oil, salt and pepper to taste. Place the salmon trout on top of the potatoes. Garnish with fresh rosemary and fresh sage. Bake in the oven for about 30 minutes, until the salmon trout is cooked and the potatoes are golden.

Nutritional values:

Calories: approximately 500 kcal

Protein: approximately 40 g

Fat: approximately 25 g

Carbohydrates: approximately 10 g

VEGETABLE ROLLS WITH FETA AND TOMATOES

Preparation time: 20 minutes

Cooking time: 15 minutes

Doses: 1 person

Ingredients:

1 medium courgette

1 medium aubergine

100 g of feta

5 cherry tomatoes

1 tablespoon of oil

extra virgin olive oil

Fresh basil

Salt and Pepper To Taste

Preparation:

Wash the courgette and aubergine and cut them into thin strips. Grill the courgette and aubergine strips for a few minutes on each side, until they are soft. Crumble the feta into a bowl. Cut the cherry tomatoes into small pieces. Mix the feta, cherry tomatoes, extra virgin olive oil, fresh basil, salt and pepper to taste. Place a spoonful of the feta and cherry tomato mixture on each strip of grilled courgette and aubergine. Roll the vegetable strips to form rolls. Serve the vegetable rolls with feta and tomatoes. **Nutritional values:**

Calories: approximately 350 kcal

Protein: approximately 30 g

Fat: approximately 20 g

Carbohydrates: approximately 5 g

LEMON CHICKEN BREAST WITH BROWN RICE

Preparation time: 20 minutes

Cooking time: 30 minutes

Doses: 1 person

Ingredients:

150 g of chicken breast

1 lemon

1 tablespoon of oil

extra virgin olive oil

Fresh rosemary

Fresh sage

Salt and Pepper To Taste

80 g of brown rice

Preparation:

Wash the chicken breast and dry it well with kitchen paper. Salt and pepper the chicken breast on both sides. In a non-stick pan, heat the extra virgin olive oil and cook the chicken breast for about 5 minutes per side, until golden and cooked. In the meantime, prepare the brown rice: rinse the rice under running water and cook it in boiling salted water for about 30 minutes, until it is soft. Serve the lemon chicken breast with brown rice, garnished with fresh rosemary and fresh sage.

Nutritional values:

Calories: approximately 450 kcal

Protein: approximately 50 g

Fat: approximately 15 g

Carbohydrates: approximately 20 g

TURKEY SCALOPPINE WITH MUSHROOMS AND PARSLEY

Preparation time: 25 minutes

Cooking time: 20 minutes

Doses: 1 person

Ingredients:

150 g of turkey slices

200 g of mixed mushrooms

1/2 small onion

1 clove of garlic

1 tablespoon of oil

extra virgin olive oil

Chopped fresh parsley

Salt and Pepper To Taste

Preparation:

Wash the turkey slices and dry them well with kitchen paper. Salt and pepper the turkey slices on both sides. In a non-stick pan, heat the extra virgin olive oil and fry the chopped onion and chopped garlic for a few minutes, until soft. Add the mixed mushrooms and cook them for about 5 minutes, stirring often. Add the turkey slices and cook them for about 5 minutes on each side, until they are golden and cooked. Add the chopped fresh parsley and mix gently. Serve the turkey escalopes with mushrooms and parsley. Nutritional values:

Calories: approximately 400 kcal

Protein: approximately 45 g

Fat: approximately 15 g

Carbohydrates: approximately 5 g

SALMON IN PAPER WITH VEGETABLES AND PESTO

Preparation time: 20 minutes

Cooking time: 20 minutes

Doses: 1 person

Ingredients:

150 g of salmon fillet

200 g of mixed vegetables (for example, courgettes, peppers, carrots)

1 tablespoon pesto

1/2 small onion

1 clove of garlic

1 tablespoon extra virgin olive oil

Chopped fresh parsley

Salt and Pepper To Taste

Preparation:

Preheat the oven to 180°C. Wash the salmon fillet and dry it well with kitchen paper. Wash the mixed vegetables and cut them into pieces. In a bowl, mix the vegetables with the extra virgin olive oil, salt and pepper to taste. Place the salmon fillet on a sheet of baking paper. Arrange the vegetables around the salmon. Add the pesto and chopped fresh parsley. Close the baking paper bag. Bake in the oven for about 20 minutes, until the salmon is cooked and the vegetables are soft.

Nutritional values:

Calories: approximately 450 kcal

Protein: approximately 45 g

Fat: approximately 20 g

Carbohydrates: approximately 5 g

CHICKPEA AND LENTIL VEGETARIAN BURGER

Preparation time: 30 minutes

Cooking time: 20 minutes

Doses: 1 person

Ingredients:

100 g of dried chickpeas

100 g of dried lentils

1 small onion

1 clove of garlic

1 carrot

1 stalk of celery

1 tablespoon breadcrumbs

1/2 teaspoon cumin

1/4 teaspoon sweet paprika

1/4 teaspoon turmeric

Salt and Pepper To Taste

Extra virgin olive oil for frying

Preparation:

Rinse the chickpeas and lentils under running water and soak them for at least 12 hours. Drain them and rinse them again. In a saucepan, cook the chickpeas and lentils in boiling water for about 30 minutes, until soft. Meanwhile, chop the onion, garlic, carrot and celery. In a non-stick pan, heat a drizzle of extra virgin olive oil and fry the chopped vegetables for a few minutes, until softened. Drain the cooked chickpeas and lentils and mash them with a fork.

Combine the chopped vegetables, breadcrumbs, cumin, sweet paprika, turmeric, salt and pepper to taste. Mix the mixture well and form two burgers. In a non-stick pan, heat a drizzle of extra virgin olive oil and cook the vegetarian burgers for about 5 minutes per side, until they are golden and cooked.

Nutritional values:

Calories: approximately 400 kcal

Protein: approximately 30 g

Fat: approximately 15 g

Carbohydrates: approximately 20 g

GRILLED BEEF FILLET WITH GRILLED VEGETABLES

Preparation time: 20 minutes

Cooking time: 15 minutes

Doses: 1 person

Ingredients:

150 g of beef fillet

200 g of mixed vegetables (for example, courgettes, peppers, aubergines)

1 tablespoon extra virgin olive oil

Fresh rosemary

Fresh sage

Salt and Pepper To Taste

Preparation:

Wash the beef fillet and dry it well with kitchen paper. Salt and pepper the beef fillet on both sides. Wash the mixed vegetables and cut them into pieces. In a non-stick pan, heat the extra virgin olive oil and grill the vegetables for a few minutes on each side, until they are soft. Grill the beef fillet for about 5 minutes per side, until browned and cooked through. Serve the grilled beef fillet with the grilled vegetables, garnished with fresh rosemary and fresh sage.

Nutritional values:

Calories: approximately 450 kcal

Protein: approximately 50 g

Fat: approximately 20 g

Carbohydrates: approximately 5 g

VEGETABLE OMELETTE WITH LIGHT CHEESE

Preparation time: 20 minutes

Cooking time: 10 minutes

Doses: 1 person

Ingredients:

2 eggs

200 g of mixed vegetables (for example, courgettes, peppers, onions)

50 g of grated light cheese

1 tablespoon extra virgin olive oil

Fresh basil

Salt and Pepper To Taste

Preparation:

Beat the eggs in a bowl with a pinch of salt. Wash the mixed vegetables and cut them into small pieces. In a non-stick pan, heat the extra virgin olive oil and fry the vegetables for a few minutes, until they are wilted. Pour the beaten eggs into the pan and mix gently. Add the grated light cheese and the chopped fresh basil. Cook the omelette for about 5 minutes, until cooked. Fold the omelette in half and serve hot.

Nutritional values:

Calories: approximately 350 kcal

Protein: approximately 30 g

Fat: approximately 15 g

Carbohydrates: approximately 5 g

SEA BASS WITH SEASONAL VEGETABLES

Preparation time: 30 minutes

Cooking time: 45 minutes

Doses: 1 person

Ingredients:

1 whole sea bass

weighing approximately 500 g

1 kg of coarse salt

200 g of seasonal vegetables (for example,

tomatoes, courgettes, potatoes)

1 tablespoon extra virgin olive oil

Chopped fresh parsley

Salt and Pepper To Taste

Preparation:

Preheat the oven to 200°C. Wash the sea bass and dry it well with kitchen paper. In a baking pan, place a layer of coarse salt. Place the sea bass on the bed of salt. Distribute the seasonal vegetables around the sea bass. Cover the sea bass with another layer of coarse salt, sealing the edges well. Bake in the oven for about 45 minutes. Remove the pan from the oven and leave to rest for a few minutes. Break the salt crust with a spoon and remove the sea bass. Remove the skin and fins of the sea bass. Flake the sea bass meat with a fork. Season the sea bass with a drizzle of extra virgin olive oil, chopped fresh parsley, salt and pepper to taste. Serve the salted sea bass with seasonal vegetables. Nutritional values:

Calories: approximately 500 kcal, Proteins: approximately 60 g

Fat: approximately 15 g, Carbohydrates: approximately 5 g

CHICKEN SCALOPPINE WITH MUSHROOMS WITH MASHED POTATOES

Preparation time: 30 minutes

Cooking time: 20 minutes

Doses: 1 person

Ingredients:

150 g of chicken breast slices

200 g of mixed mushrooms

1/2 small onion

1 clove of garlic

1 tablespoon extra virgin olive oil

Chopped fresh parsley

Salt and Pepper To Taste

200 g of potatoes

Skimmed milk to taste

Preparation:

Wash the chicken breast slices and dry them well with kitchen paper. Salt and pepper the chicken breast slices on both sides. In a non-stick pan, heat the extra virgin olive oil and fry the chopped onion and chopped garlic for a few minutes, until soft. Add the mixed mushrooms and cook them for about 5 minutes, stirring often. Add the chicken breast slices and cook them for about 5 minutes per side, until they are golden and cooked. Meanwhile, prepare the mashed potatoes: peel the potatoes and cut them into pieces.

Cook the potatoes in boiling salted water for about 15 minutes, until they are soft. Mash the potatoes with a fork and add a little skimmed milk to obtain a creamy mixture. Serve the chicken cutlets with mushrooms with the mashed potatoes, garnished with chopped fresh parsley. Nutritional values:

Calories: approximately 550 kcal

Protein: approximately 50 g

Fat: approximately 20 g

Carbohydrates: approximately 30 g

TURKEY BURGER WITH WHEEL BREAD AND GRILLED VEGETABLES

Preparation time: 25 minutes

Cooking time: 20 minutes

Doses: 1 person

Ingredients:

150 g of minced turkey

1 wholemeal sandwich

1/2 small onion

1 tomato

1 courgette

1 aubergine

1 tablespoon extra virgin olive oil

Chopped fresh parsley

Salt and Pepper To Taste

Preparation:

Wash the courgette and aubergine and cut them into slices. Grill the courgette and aubergine slices for a few minutes on each side, until they are soft. In a non-stick pan, heat the extra virgin olive oil and fry the chopped onion for a few minutes, until it softens. Add the ground turkey and cook it by crumbling it with a wooden spoon for about 5 minutes, until it is browned. Salt and pepper the turkey mixture. Heat the wholemeal sandwich. Assemble the hamburger: spread a little chopped fresh parsley on the wholemeal bun, add the turkey mixture, the tomato slices and the grilled courgette and aubergine slices. Close the sandwich and serve the turkey burger with grilled vegetables. Nutritional values:

Calories: approximately 450 kcal, Protein: approximately 40 g

Fat: approximately 15 g, Carbohydrates: approximately 20 g

SALMON FILLET IN PISTACHIO CRUST WITH WHOLE WHOLE COUS COUS

Preparation time: 30 minutes

Cooking time: 25 minutes

Doses: 1 person

Ingredients:

150 g of salmon fillet

50 g of chopped pistachios

2 tablespoons of breadcrumbs

1 tablespoon extra virgin olive oil

Chopped fresh parsley

Salt and Pepper To Taste

80 g of wholemeal couscous

Vegetable broth to taste

Preparation:

Preheat the oven to 200°C.

Wash the salmon fillet and dry it well with kitchen paper. In a bowl, mix the chopped pistachios, breadcrumbs, extra virgin olive oil, chopped fresh parsley, salt and pepper to taste. Spread the pistachio mixture over the salmon fillet. Arrange the pistachio crusted salmon fillet on a baking tray lined with baking paper. Bake in the oven for about 20 minutes, until the salmon is cooked and the crust is golden. In the meantime, prepare the wholemeal couscous: in a pan, bring the vegetable broth to the boil. Remove from the heat and add the wholemeal couscous. Cover the pan with a cloth and leave to rest for about 5 minutes. Fluff the whole couscous with a fork. Serve the salmon fillet in a pistachio crust with the wholemeal couscous. Nutritional values:

Calories: approximately 500 kcal, Proteins: approximately 45 g

Fat: approximately 20 g, Carbohydrates: approximately 30 g

BEEF STEAK WITH GRILLED PEPPERS

Preparation time: 20 minutes

Cooking time: 20 minutes

Doses: 1 person

Ingredients:

150 g of beef steak

2 peppers

1 tablespoon of oil

extra virgin olive oil

Fresh rosemary

Fresh sage

Salt and Pepper To Taste

Preparation:

Wash the beef steak and dry it well with kitchen paper. Salt and pepper the beef steak on both sides. Wash the peppers and cut them into slices. Grill the sirloin steak for about 5 minutes per side, until cooked through. Grill the peppers for about 10 minutes, until soft. Serve the sirloin steak with the grilled peppers, garnished with fresh rosemary and fresh sage.

Nutritional values:

Calories: approximately 450 kcal

Protein: approximately 50 g

Fat: approximately 20 g

Carbohydrates: approximately 5 g

AUBERGINES ROLLS WITH VEGETABLES AND LIGHT CHEESE

Preparation time: 30 minutes

Cooking time: 20 minutes

Doses: 1 person

Ingredients:

1 aubergine

100 g of courgette

50 g of grated light cheese

1 tablespoon of oil

extra virgin olive oil

Fresh basil

Salt and Pepper To Taste

Preparation:

Wash the aubergine and cut it into thin slices. Grill the aubergine slices for a few minutes on each side, until they are softened. Wash the courgettes and cut them into strips. In a non-stick pan, heat the extra virgin olive oil and fry the courgettes for a few minutes, until they are soft. Add the grated light cheese and the chopped fresh basil, mixing well. Place a spoonful of the zucchini and cheese mixture on each slice of grilled aubergine. Roll the aubergine slices to form rolls. Serve the aubergine rolls with vegetables and light cheese. Nutritional values:

Calories: approximately 350 kcal, Protein: approximately 30 g

Fat: approximately 15 g, Carbohydrates: approximately 5 g

SLICED BEEF WITH MIXED SALAD AND SEASONED TOMATOES

Preparation time: 20 minutes

Cooking time: 15 minutes

Doses: 1 person

Ingredients:

200 g of cut beef

100 g of mixed salad

(lettuce, rocket, valerian)

10 cherry tomatoes

1 tablespoon extra virgin olive oil

Balsamic vinegar to taste

Salt and Pepper To Taste

Preparation:

Grill the beef steak for about 5 minutes per side, until cooked to your liking. Wash the mixed salad and cut it into pieces. Wash the cherry tomatoes and cut them in half. In a bowl, season the mixed salad with extra virgin olive oil, balsamic vinegar, salt and pepper to taste. Arrange the mixed salad on a serving plate. Slice the beef steak and arrange it over the salad. Decorate with the seasoned cherry tomatoes.

Nutritional values:

Calories: approximately 500 kcal

Protein: approximately 60 g

Fat: approximately 20 g

Carbohydrates: approximately 5 g

SWORDFISH WITH LEMON WITH BULGUR AND VEGETABLES

Preparation time: 30 minutes

Cooking time: 20 minutes

Doses: 1 person

Ingredients:

200 g of swordfish

80 g of bulgur

100 g of mixed vegetables (for example, courgettes, peppers, onions)

1 tablespoon extra virgin olive oil

Juice of 1 lemon

Chopped fresh parsley

Salt and Pepper To Taste

Preparation:

Cook the bulgur in boiling salted water for about 15 minutes, until soft. Wash the swordfish and cut it into slices. Wash the mixed vegetables and cut them into small pieces. In a non-stick pan, heat the extra virgin olive oil and fry the vegetables for a few minutes, until they are wilted. Add the swordfish steaks and cook them for about 5 minutes on each side, until they are cooked. Add the lemon juice and cook for another minute. Drain the bulgur and add it to the vegetables and swordfish. Season with chopped fresh parsley, salt and pepper to taste. Nutritional values:

Calories: approximately 450 kcal

Protein: approximately 50 g

Fat: approximately 15 g

Carbohydrates: approximately 20 g

SIDE DISH RECIPES

CUCUMBER AND TOMATO SALAD WITH APPLE VINEGAR AND AROMATIC HERBS

Preparation time: 15 minutes

Cooking time: -

Doses: 1 person

Ingredients:

1 medium cucumber

1 medium tomato

1 tablespoon extra virgin olive oil

1 tablespoon apple cider vinegar

1/2 teaspoon dried oregano

1/4 teaspoon dried thyme

Salt and Pepper To Taste

Preparation:

Wash the cucumber and tomato. Cut the cucumber into thin slices and the tomato into cubes. In a bowl, mix the cucumber, tomato, extra virgin olive oil, apple cider vinegar, dried oregano, dried thyme, salt and pepper to taste. Serve the fresh cucumber and tomato salad.

Nutritional values:

Calories: approximately 150 kcal

Protein: approximately 2 g

Fat: approximately 10 g

Carbohydrates: approximately 5 g

GRILLED ASPARAGUS WITH OLIVE OIL AND BLACK PEPPER

Preparation time: 10 minutes

Cooking time: 10 minutes

Doses: 1 person

Ingredients:

150 g of asparagus

1 tablespoon of oil

extra virgin olive oil

Black pepper to taste

Preparation:

Wash the asparagus and cut the hard end part. Grill the asparagus for about 10 minutes, turning often, until tender. Season the grilled asparagus with extra virgin olive oil and black pepper to taste. Serve the grilled asparagus hot.

Nutritional values:

Calories: approximately 100 kcal

Protein: approximately 3 g

Fat: approximately 8 g

Carbohydrates: approximately 3 g

SAUTÉED CHAMPIGNON MUSHROOMS WITH GARLIC AND PARSLEY

Preparation time: 15 minutes

Cooking time: 10 minutes

Doses: 1 person

Ingredients:

200 g of champignon mushrooms

1 clove of garlic

1 tablespoon of oil

extra virgin olive oil

Chopped fresh parsley

Salt and Pepper To Taste

Preparation:

Wash the champignon mushrooms and cut them into slices. In a non-stick pan, heat the extra virgin olive oil and fry the chopped garlic for a minute. Add the button mushrooms and cook them for about 10 minutes, stirring often, until they are tender. Season the sautéed champignon mushrooms with chopped fresh parsley, salt and pepper to taste. Serve the sautéed champignon mushrooms hot.

Nutritional values:

Calories: approximately 150 kcal

Protein: approximately 3 g

Fat: approximately 10 g

Carbohydrates: approximately 5 g

GRILLED COURGETTES WITH PEPPERS AND ONIONS

Preparation time: 20 minutes

Cooking time: 20 minutes

Doses: 1 person

Ingredients:

1 medium courgette

1/2 bell pepper

1/2 onion

1 tablespoon of oil

extra virgin olive oil

Dried oregano to taste

Salt and Pepper To Taste

Preparation:

Wash the courgette, pepper and onion. Cut the courgette into slices, the pepper into strips and the onion into rings. Grill the vegetables for about 10 minutes per side, until soft. Season the grilled vegetables with extra virgin olive oil, dried oregano, salt and pepper to taste. Serve the grilled vegetables hot.

Nutritional values:

Calories: approximately 150 kcal

Protein: approximately 2 g

Fat: approximately 10 g

Carbohydrates: approximately 5 g

BAKED AUBERGINES WITH TOMATO AND BASIL SAUCE

Preparation time: 30 minutes

Cooking time: 30 minutes

Doses: 1 person

Ingredients:

1 medium aubergine

200 g of tomato sauce

Fresh basil

Extra virgin olive oil to taste

Salt and Pepper To Taste

Preparation:

Preheat the oven to 180°C. Wash the aubergine and cut it into slices. Arrange the aubergine slices on a baking tray lined with baking paper. Season the aubergines with extra virgin olive oil, salt and pepper to taste. Pour the tomato sauce over the aubergines. Bake in the oven for about 30 minutes, until the aubergines are soft. Garnish with fresh basil leaves. Serve the baked aubergines with hot tomato and basil sauce.

Nutritional values:

Calories: approximately 250 kcal

Protein: approximately 8 g

Fat: approximately 15 g

Carbohydrates: approximately 10 g

MIXED SALAD WITH CHYCORY, LETTUCE, ARUGULA AND GRATED CARROTS

Preparation time: 10 minutes

Cooking time: -

Doses: 1 person

Ingredients:

50 g of Chicory

50 g of Lettuce

30 g of Arugula

1 medium carrot

1 tablespoon of oil

extra virgin olive oil

Lemon juice to taste

Salt and Pepper To Taste

Preparation:

Wash the Chicory, lettuce and Arugula. Cut the Chicory into strips and the lettuce into leaves. Grate the carrot. In a bowl, mix the Chicory, lettuce, Arugula, grated carrot, extra virgin olive oil, lemon juice, salt and pepper to taste. You can add other vegetables of your choice to the grilled vegetables, such as tomatoes or mushrooms.

Serve the fresh mixed salad.

Nutritional values:

Calories: approximately 100 kcal

Protein: approximately 3 g

Fat: approximately 5 g

Carbohydrates: approximately 5 g

COLD QUINOA WITH PEPPERS, TOMATOES AND BLACK OLIVES

Preparation time: 20 minutes

Cooking time: 15 minutes

Doses: 1 person

Ingredients:

80 g of quinoa

1/2 bell pepper

10 cherry tomatoes

10 black olives

1 tablespoon of oil

extra virgin olive oil

Dried oregano to taste

Salt and Pepper To Taste

Preparation:

Cook the quinoa in boiling salted water for about 15 minutes, until cooked. Wash the pepper and cut it into small pieces. Wash the cherry tomatoes and cut them in half. Drain the quinoa and season it with extra virgin olive oil, salt and pepper to taste. Add the bell pepper, cherry tomatoes and black olives to the quinoa. Mix well and leave to rest in the refrigerator for at least 30 minutes before serving.

Nutritional values:

Calories: approximately 350 kcal

Protein: approximately 15 g

Fat: approximately 15 g

Carbohydrates: approximately 30 g

BAKED SWEET POTATOES WITH ROSEMARY AND GARLIC

Preparation time: 15 minutes

Cooking time: 45 minutes

Doses: 1 person

Ingredients:

1 medium sweet potato

1 clove of garlic

1 sprig of rosemary

1 tablespoon of oil

extra virgin olive oil

Salt and Pepper To Taste

Preparation:

Preheat the oven to 200°C. Wash the sweet potato and peel it. Cut the sweet potato into slices about 1cm thick. Arrange the sweet potato slices on a baking tray lined with baking paper. Season the sweet potatoes with extra virgin olive oil, salt and pepper to taste. Add the chopped garlic and the rosemary sprig. Bake for about 45 minutes, until the sweet potatoes are soft.

Nutritional values:

Calories: approximately 200 kcal

Protein: approximately 2 g

Fat: approximately 10 g

Carbohydrates: approximately 30 g

COURGETTE FLAN WITH RICOTTA AND EGGS

Preparation time: 20 minutes

Cooking time: 30 minutes

Doses: 1 person

Ingredients:

200 g of courgettes

100 g of ricotta

2 eggs

2 tablespoons of

grated Parmesan cheese

Salt and Pepper To Taste

Preparation:

Wash the courgettes and grate them. In a bowl, mix the grated courgettes, ricotta, eggs, grated parmesan, salt and pepper to taste. Pour the mixture onto a baking tray lined with baking paper. Bake in the oven at 180°C for about 30 minutes, until the flan is golden. You can add other ingredients of your choice to the cold quinoa, such as feta, corn or chickpeas. You can use another type of herb for baked sweet potatoes, such as thyme or sage. If you prefer, you can cook the courgette flan in a pan over low heat for about 20 minutes. Nutritional values:

Calories: approximately 250 kcal

Protein: approximately 20 g

Fat: approximately 15 g

Carbohydrates: approximately 5 g

WHOLE WHOLE COUS COUS WITH GRILLED VEGETABLES AND FRESH MINT

Preparation time: 20 minutes

Cooking time: 10 minutes

Doses: 1 person

Ingredients:

80 g of wholemeal couscous

1 medium courgette

1/2 bell pepper

1 red onion

1 tablespoon of oil

extra virgin olive oil

Fresh mint to taste

Salt and Pepper To Taste

Preparation:

Cook the wholemeal couscous in boiling salted water for about 10 minutes, until cooked. Wash the courgette, pepper and red onion. Cut the courgette into slices, the pepper into strips and the onion into rings. Grill the vegetables for about 10 minutes per side, until soft. Drain the wholemeal couscous and season it with extra virgin olive oil, salt and pepper to taste. Add the grilled vegetables to the couscous and mix well. Garnish with fresh mint leaves. Serve the wholemeal couscous with grilled vegetables and warm fresh mint.

Nutritional values:

Calories: approximately 350 kcal

Protein: approximately 15 g

Fat: approximately 15 g

Carbohydrates: approximately 30 g

BAKED POTATOES WITH ROSEMARY AND GARLIC

Preparation time: 15 minutes

Cooking time: 45 minutes

Doses: 1 person

Ingredients:

1 medium potato

1 clove of garlic

1 sprig of rosemary

1 tablespoon of oil

extra virgin olive oil

Salt and Pepper To Taste

Preparation:

Preheat the oven to 200°C. Wash the potato and peel it. Cut the potato into slices about 1 cm thick. Arrange the potato slices on a baking tray lined with baking paper. Season the potatoes with extra virgin olive oil, salt and pepper to taste. Add the chopped garlic and the rosemary sprig. Bake in the oven for about 45 minutes, until the potatoes are soft.

Nutritional values:

Calories: approximately 200 kcal

Protein: approximately 2 g

Fat: approximately 10 g

Carbohydrates: approximately 30 g

MIXED VEGETABLE OMELETTE WITH SPINACH, TOMATOES AND COURGETTES

Preparation time: 20 minutes

Cooking time: 15 minutes

Doses: 1 person

Ingredients:

2 eggs

50 g of spinach

5 cherry tomatoes

1/2 courgette

1 tablespoon of oil

extra virgin olive oil

Salt and Pepper To Taste

Preparation:

Wash the spinach, cherry tomatoes and courgette. Fry the chopped courgette in a non-stick pan with a spoonful of extra virgin olive oil for a couple of minutes. Add the spinach and cook for another minute, until wilted. Add the cherry tomatoes cut in half and cook for a minute. In a bowl, beat the eggs with a pinch of salt and pepper. Pour the egg mixture into the pan with the vegetables and cook over low heat for about 10 minutes, until the omelette is cooked. Fold the omelette in half and serve hot.

Nutritional values:

Calories: approximately 250 kcal

Protein: approximately 20 g

Fat: approximately 15 g

Carbohydrates: approximately 5 g

CONCLUSION

As we conclude our journey together through the Dukan Diet 2025, I sincerely hope that you have found inspiration, motivation, and most importantly, tangible results on your journey to wellness and your desired weight. I kindly invite you to share your experience and feedback about this book. Reviews are critical to helping other readers discover the value of this program and to supporting the author's work. If you enjoyed the book and it had a positive impact on your life, I would be extremely grateful if you could take a few minutes of your time to leave a review. Your opinion matters and can make a difference to those looking for reliable guidance in their quest for health and wellness.

Thank you for dedicating your time and attention to these pages, for showing a sincere interest in understanding and improving your health. Your words could be a guiding light for other wellness seekers embarking on this path. I thank you deeply for choosing The Dukan Diet 2025. Thank you very much for choosing to accompany me on this journey and for investing in your health and well-being. I wish you all the success and happiness in your future journey.With gratitude, KLARLOCK